Pediatric Colorectal and Pelvic Surgery

Case Studies

Pediatric Colorectal and Pelvic Surgery
Case Studies

Victoria A. Lane, MBChB, MRCS
Nationwide Children's Hospital
Columbus, Ohio, USA

Leeds Children's Hospital, Leeds General Infirmary
Leeds, United Kingdom

Richard J. Wood, MD
Nationwide Children's Hospital
The Ohio State University College of Medicine
Columbus, Ohio, USA

Carlos A. Reck-Burneo, MD
Nationwide Children's Hospital
Columbus, Ohio, USA

Medical University of Vienna
General Hospital Vienna (AKH)
Vienna, Austria

Marc A. Levitt, MD
Nationwide Children's Hospital
The Ohio State University College of Medicine
Columbus, Ohio, USA

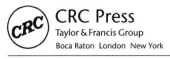

CRC Press
Taylor & Francis Group
Boca Raton London New York

CRC Press is an imprint of the
Taylor & Francis Group, an **informa** business

CRC Press
Taylor & Francis Group
6000 Broken Sound Parkway NW, Suite 300
Boca Raton, FL 33487-2742

© 2017 by Taylor & Francis Group, LLC
CRC Press is an imprint of Taylor & Francis Group, an Informa business

International Standard Book Number-13: 978-1-1380-3177-7 (Pack- Hardback and Ebook)

Visit the Taylor & Francis Web site at
http://www.taylorandfrancis.com

and the CRC Press Web site at
http://www.crcpress.com

Contents

Foreword

It is indeed an honor and a pleasure for me to write the foreword to our son Marc's book written with his colleagues Victoria Lane, Carlos Reck, and Richard Wood. Marc has indicated that the case-based teaching method that I have used with my co-author, Howard Weiner, since 1971, for *Neurology for the House Officer* (translated into eight foreign languages), *Case Studies in Neurology for the House Officer,* and in our annual neurology course served as a stimulus for the current endeavor. Over a cumulative 70 years of teaching, we found that teaching by specific illustrative cases was the most effective method for producing lasting retention of clinical knowledge. I hope that this book proves helpful in educating other pediatric caregivers, but most importantly that it helps solve pediatric colorectal and pelvic surgical problems in children from all over the world.

Lawrence P. Levitt, MD
Professor Emeritus of Neurology
Lehigh Valley Hospital, Allentown, PA, USA

Preface

The book is intended to teach the key principles in the management of colorectal and pelvic diagnoses through case-based presentations. We believe it will be valuable for all members of the management team that cares for children with these problems, including the surgeon, the pediatrician, the gastroenterologist, the neonatologist, the nurse, the pediatric surgical trainee, and the medical student.

The book encompasses the wide range of complex colorectal issues, including:

- Primary diagnosis, management, radiology, and histopathology of Hirschsprung disease
- Primary diagnosis, management, and radiology of anorectal malformations
- Bowel management for fecal incontinence in a variety of patient groups
- The problematic post-operative Hirschsprung disease, and anorectal malformation
- Operative techniques including pitfalls and challenges

We hope that this book will serve as an educational tool for those treating children with colorectal and pelvic problems and will therefore help to improve the care provided and reduce the morbidity seen in this group of patients.

And, to our families for their tireless support, devotion, and love—we thank you.

Victoria A. Lane
Richard J. Wood
Carlos A. Reck-Burneo
Marc A. Levitt

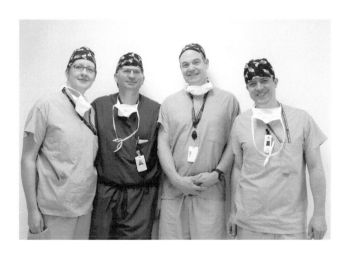

Contributors

We are grateful to the colleagues listed below for their contributions to this book.

Abbey Ballard, RN, BSN
Center for Colorectal and Pelvic Reconstruction
Nationwide Children's Hospital
Columbus, Ohio

D. Gregory Bates, MD
Assistant Chief and Chief of Clinical Operations
Department of Radiology
Children's Hospital and Children's Radiological
    Institute
Clinical Associate Professor of Radiology
The Ohio State University College of Medicine and
    Public Health
Columbus, Ohio

Ashley Bober, RN, BSN
Center for Colorectal and Pelvic Reconstruction
Nationwide Children's Hospital
Columbus, Ohio

Julie Choueiki, MSN, RN, CPEN
Center for Colorectal and Pelvic Reconstruction
Nationwide Children's Hospital
Columbus, Ohio

Onnalisa Nash, MSN, CPNP
Center for Colorectal and Pelvic Reconstruction
Nationwide Children's Hospital
Columbus, Ohio

Kaleigh B. Peters, MS, APN, NP-C
Center for Colorectal and Pelvic Reconstruction
Nationwide Children's Hospital
Columbus, Ohio

Meghan Peters, RN, BSN
Center for Colorectal and Pelvic Reconstruction
Nationwide Children's Hospital
Columbus, Ohio

Vinay Prasad, MD, FASCP, FCAP
Director of Surgical Pathology
Director of Pediatric GI Pathology
Nationwide Children's Hospital
Columbus, Ohio

Clare Skerritt, MBBS, MSc, MRCS (England)
Pediatric Surgical Registrar
Evelina London Children's Hospital
London, United Kingdom

Stephanie Vyrostek, RN, BSN
Center for Colorectal and Pelvic Reconstruction
Nationwide Children's Hospital
Columbus, Ohio

Andrea Wagner, MS, CPNP
Center for Colorectal and Pelvic Reconstruction
Nationwide Children's Hospital
Columbus, Ohio

Acknowledgements

We are grateful to the colleagues listed below for the support they provide in the care of patients, their individual roles on our wonderful and collaborative team, and their help in organizing a variety of aspects of this book.

- Katrina Abram
- Brent Adler
- Shumyle Alam
- Alyssa Albany
- Charmaign Albright
- Jennifer Aldrink
- Steve Allen
- Seth Alpert
- James Anderson
- Steve Anderson
- Jeff Avansino
- Andrew Banks
- Jillean Bastian
- Becky Batka
- Rachael Bellisari
- Janet Berry
- Gail Besner
- Kristina Booth
- Lesley Breech
- Morris Brown
- Rich Brilli
- Laura Brubaker
- Amy Byer
- Roberta Chaney
- Nicole Chave
- Christina Ching
- Marissa Condon
- Ted Copetas
- Kristine Creviston
- Jackie Cronau
- Daniel DaJusta
- Katherine Deans
- Ivo Deblaauw
- Belinda Dickie
- Karen Diefenbach
- Carlo DiLorenzo
- Robert Dyckes
- Morris Brown

- Lesley Breech
- Pam Edson
- Christine Frake
- Jeremy Fisher
- Jason Frischer
- Molly Fuchs
- Aaron Garrison
- Alessandra Gasior
- Julie Gerberick
- Rashaun Geter
- Dani Gonzalez
- Jamie Goodall
- Keysha Hancock
- Andria Haynes
- Meg Heischman
- Karen Heiser
- Michael Helmrath
- Andrea Hetrick
- Geri Hewitt
- Connie Hieatt
- Ann Hoffman
- Jennie Hoffman
- Stuart Hosie
- Denise Howe
- Venkata R. Jayanthi
- Laura Keibler
- Lorraine Kelley-Quon
- Andrea Kesar
- Avery Kondik
- Jennifer Kondik
- Steve Kraus
- Martin Lacher
- Diane Lang
- Jack Langer
- Timothy Lee
- Stacie Leeper
- Nelson Lees
- Jeffrey Leonard

- Vickie Leonhardt
- Eva Levitt
- Ernesto Levy
- Peter Lu
- Carol Maynard
- Kate McCracken
- Emily McDowell
- Daryl McLeod
- Marc Michalsky
- Paola Midrio
- Rick Miller
- Pete Minneci
- Dennis Minzler
- Mary Lee Montgomery
- Larry Moss
- Erin Ney
- Alp Numanoglu
- Kim Osborne
- Kathy Pazaropoulos
- Allison Pegg
- Gil Peri
- Jeb Phillips
- Ron Pontius
- Leah Reilly
- Stephanie Riesenberg
- Tim Robinson
- Michael Rollins
- Brenda Ruth
- Payam Saadai
- Danielle Sabol
- Stephen Sales
- Alejandra Vilanova Sanchez
- Christine Sander
- Ashley Sanders
- Miguel Saps
- Sabine Sarnecki
- Alicia Shoemaker
- Dipali Sitapara

- Pim Sloots
- Seryna Smith
- Tara Smith
- Eric Sribnick
- Ian Sugarman
- Jonathan Sutcliffe
- Heather Tackett
- Stephen Testa
- Raj Thakkar

- Benjamin Thompson
- Mandy Thompson
- Bethanne Tilson
- Katherine Toadvine
- Kathleen Tucker
- Anna Varughese
- Karla Vaz
- Laura Weaver
- Renee Carpenter Wells

- Chris Westgarth-Taylor
- Kara Wheeler
- Erin Willet
- Charae Williams
- Kent Williams
- Kelly Williamson
- Linda Wilson
- David Wise
- Desalegn Yacob

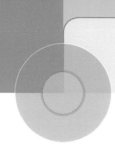

Anorectal malformations (ARM) and the ARM continence index

INTRODUCTION

Over the last 20–30 years, there have been significant advances in the management of children with anorectal malformations, both medical and surgical. Changes have also occurred in the terminology used to describe the various types of anorectal malformation. Previously, the terms "low," "intermediate," and "high" malformations were used; however, these terms are not as anatomically clear as those used in the **Krickenbeck Classification**, developed in 2005.

It is vital that the pediatric surgical community speaks the "same language" around the world, because having the correct diagnosis from the outset ensures that correct decisions can be made with regards to surgical planning and, ultimately, operative repair. In addition, accurate anatomic classification helps with the prediction of functional outcome.

Failure to recognize the type of malformation can lead to adverse results. Therefore, we must ensure that data are reported in a standardized, uniform way in order for results to be comparable.

KRICKENBECK CLASSIFICATION

Common malformations	Rare malformations
Perineal fistula	Pouch colon atresia/stenosis
Rectourethral fistula (prostatic, bulbar, bladder neck)	Rectal atresia/stenosis
Rectovesical fistula	Rectovaginal fistula
Vestibular fistula	H-type fistula
Cloaca	Others (e.g., posterior cloaca variant, cloacal exstrophy, covered cloacal exstrophy)
No fistula	
Anal stenosis	

ARM CONTINENCE INDEX

Children with anorectal malformations often have impaired functional outcomes. It is recognized that the following features are likely to impact the likelihood of the child achieving fecal continence:

- Type of anorectal malformation
- Sacral ratio
- Associated spinal anomalies

Individual components have been studied and reported in the literature. The extent to which all of these factors interact with each other (ARM continence index) is not known, but is currently under investigation.

With the development of this index, we believe that our ability to predict the likelihood of fecal continence, even prior to surgical intervention, will be improved, and that this will serve as an important guide when counseling families and setting expectations for the future.

In addition, benchmarking outcomes based on a set of parameters (type of ARM, sacral ratio and spinal anomalies) is potentially an important tool to ensuring minimum quality standards and improving the quality of care overall.

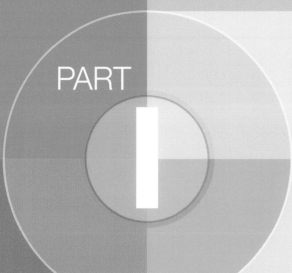

PART

I

ANORECTAL MALFORMATIONS— PRIMARY

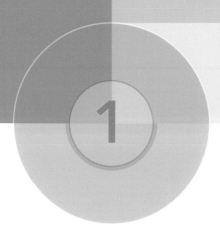

Diagnosis of an anorectal malformation

1

EXPLANATORY CHAPTER—HOW TO MAKE THE CORRECT ANATOMIC DIAGNOSIS

- Establishing the diagnosis/type of anorectal malformation (ARM) that the infant has is the most important first step when managing a child, after initial resuscitation and basic care.
- Without a clear understanding of the defect, it is impossible to make informed decisions with regards to the ongoing needs of the child.

MALE ARM

The male ARM patient can have:

- Perineal fistula
- Rectourethral fistula
    - Bulbar, prostatic, bladder neck which correspond to levels of the fistula to the urinary tract
- Recto-bladder fistula (bladder dome)
- No fistula
- Anal or rectal stenosis
- Rectal atresia
- Cloacal exstrophy

The diagnosis can be made on simple clinical examination in the majority of cases. The more complex malformations will require further investigations before one can identify the type of ARM the male infant has.

PERINEAL FISTULA

- The rectum is seen to form a fistulous tract to the perineum, anterior to the anal dimple.
- There is no communication with the urinary tract.
- The anterior rectum abuts the posterior urethra.
- Meconium (or mucous beads) will be seen on the perineum.
- Meconium is seen to be running along a fistulous tract along the midline raphe of the scrotum.
- The fistulous tract starts anterior to where the positioned anus should be.

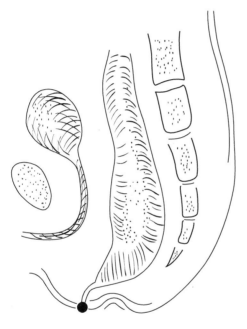

Figure 1.1 Perineal fistula.

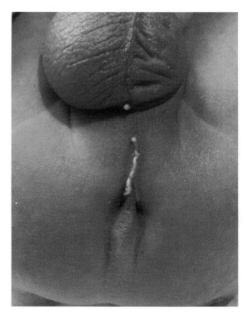

Figure 1.2 Perineal fistula.

PERINEAL FISTULA

- There is mucous from the fistula running along the midline raphe of the scrotum.
- The fistulous opening is anterior to the correct location of the anus.

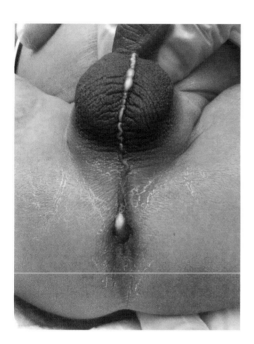

Figure 1.3 Perineal fistula.

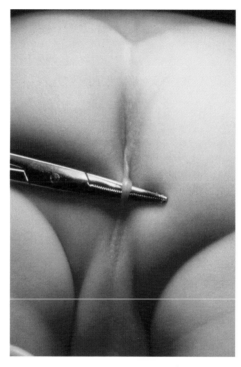

Figure 1.4 Bucket handle. Patient is in prone position. There is a "bucket handle" deformity, associated with a perineal fistula.

ANATOMY OF THE URETHRA

The urethra can be divided into:

- Penile
- Bulbar
- Prostatic
- The point of insertion of the fistula into the male urethra establishes the type of anorectal malformation.
- The exact point of insertion, however, can only be established through a distal colostogram *after* the child has had formation of a divided proximal sigmoid colostomy and mucous fistula.

RECTOURETHRAL FISTULA

- There is meconium seen at the tip of the penis indicating that there is a communication with the urinary tract.
- It is *not* possible to establish where precisely the fistula is entering the urinary tract at this stage.
- This child requires a divided proximal sigmoid colostomy with mucous fistula. Further imaging is needed to establish the exact type of anorectal malformation.

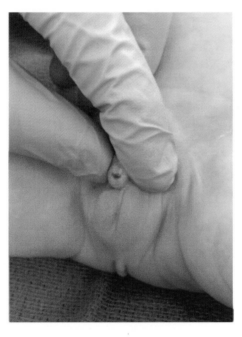

Figure 1.5 Rectourethral fistula.

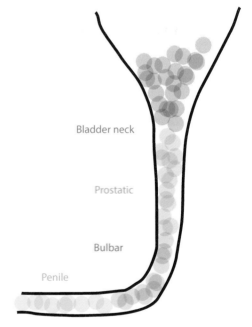

Figure 1.6 Anatomy of the urethra.

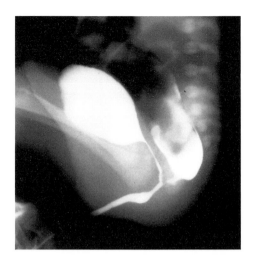

Figure 1.7 Rectobulbar fistula.

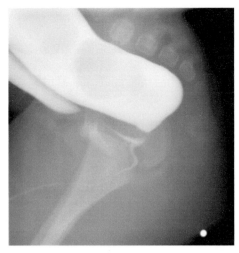

Figure 1.9 Rectoprostatic fistula.

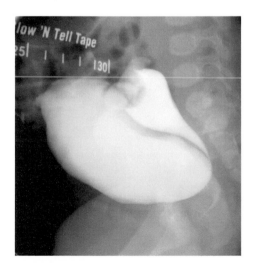

Figure 1.8 Recto-bladder neck fistula.

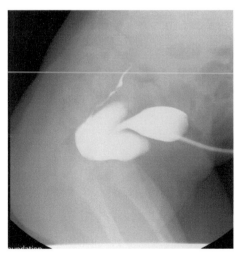

Figure 1.10 Recto-bladder fistula.

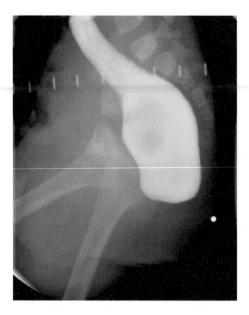

Figure 1.11 No fistula. The rectum is bulging under the pressure of the contrast being instilled (high-pressure colostogram), confirming that there is no fistula.

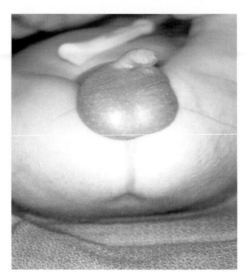

Figure 1.12 No fistula. On rare occasions, there will be no communication with the urinary tract. This is more commonly seen with trisomy 21.

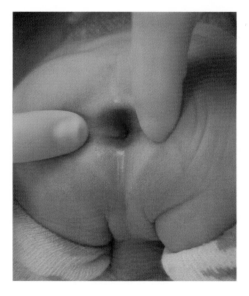

Figure 1.13 Rectal atresia. Well-centered anus in the middle of the sphincter complex. Funnel-like skin lined and blind ending.

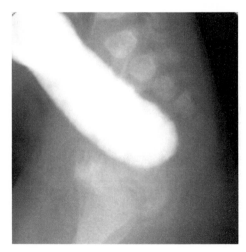

Figure 1.14 Rectal atresia.

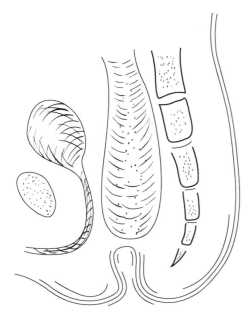

Figure 1.15 Rectal atresia.

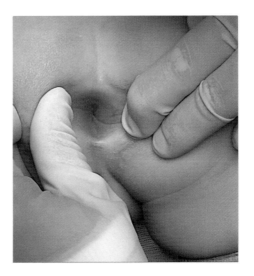

Figure 1.16 Anal stenosis. Well-centered anus in the middle of the sphincter complex, but stenotic.

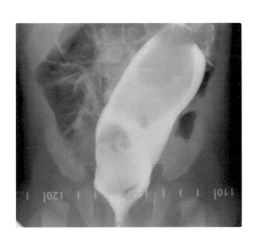

Figure 1.17 Anal stenosis.

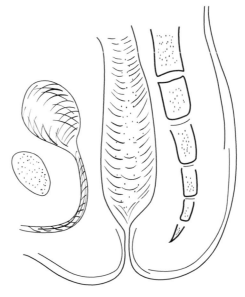

Figure 1.18 Anal stenosis.

FEMALE ANORECTAL MALFORMATIONS

The female ARM patient can have:

- Perineal fistula
- Rectovestibular fistula
- Rectal atresia/stenosis
- Cloaca
  - Short common channel (<3 cm)
  - Long common channel (>3 cm)
- Posterior cloacal variant
- Rectovaginal fistula
- Rectovesical fistula
- H-type fistula
- Cloacal exstrophy

MAKING THE DIAGNOSIS

The first place to start when attempting to make the correct diagnosis in a female is to establish how many openings there are in the perineum, and this requires careful examination.

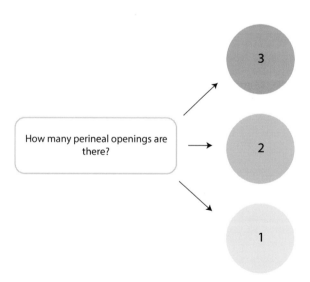

Figure 1.19 Number of perineal openings.

PERINEAL FISTULA

In this case: *Three* openings.

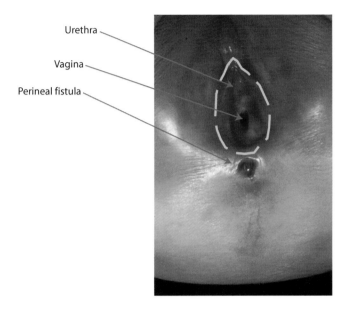

Urethra

Vagina

Perineal fistula

Figure 1.20 Perineal fistula.

RECTOVESTIBULAR FISTULA

In this case: *Three* openings.

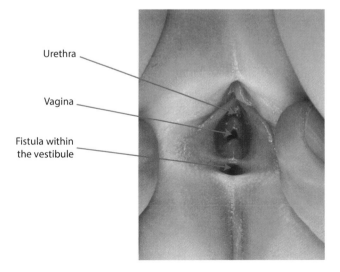

Urethra

Vagina

Fistula within
the vestibule

Figure 1.21 Rectovestibular fistula.

H-TYPE RECTOVAGINAL FISTULA

- The fistulous tract is demonstrated by the lacrimal probe.
- The urethral, vaginal, and anal openings are normal. However, there is an abnormal communication between the vagina (vestibule) and the anus (anal crypt of the dentate line).

In this case: *Three* openings.

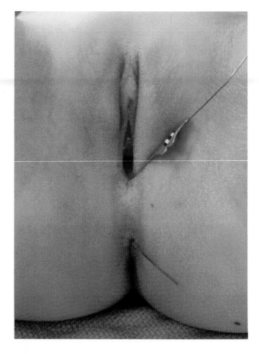

Figure 1.22 H-type rectovaginal fistula.

VAGINAL ATRESIA

- Urethra is present.
- Absent vagina.
- Rectum is present.

In this case: *Two* openings.

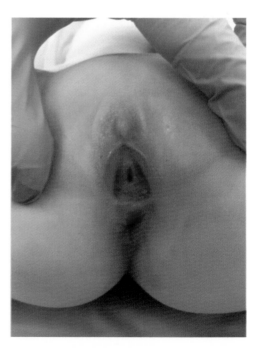

Figure 1.23 Vaginal atresia.

RECTOVAGINAL FISTULA

- Urethra.
- The fistula is opening into the posterior aspect of the vagina.
- No anus.

In this case: *Two* openings.

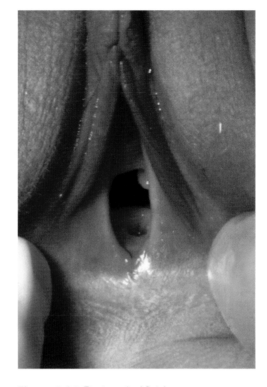

Figure 1.24 Rectovaginal fistula.

CLOACA

- There is only one opening identified in the perineum.
- There is no anal opening.

In this case: *One* opening.

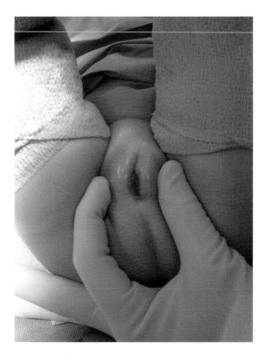

Figure 1.25 Cloaca.

CLOACA

- *Short common channel.*
- Single opening identified in the perineum.
- Common channel is <3 cm.

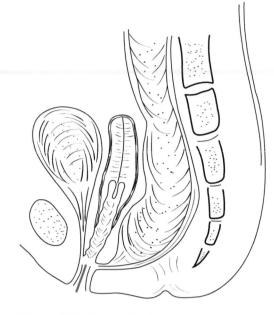

Figure 1.26 Cloaca—short common channel.

CLOACA

- *Long common channel.*
- Single opening identified in the perineum.
- Common channel is >3 cm.
- The vagina is also short and the length of the urethra to the bladder neck also needs to be assessed.

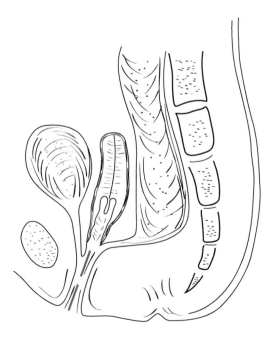

Figure 1.27 Cloaca—long common channel.

THE SACRAL RATIO

CALCULATION

Sacral ratio = YZ/XY

The lateral view for calculating the sacral ratio is more accurate

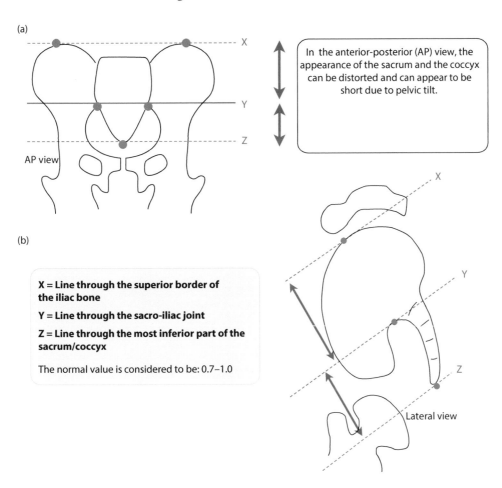

(a)

In the anterior-posterior (AP) view, the appearance of the sacrum and the coccyx can be distorted and can appear to be short due to pelvic tilt.

(b)

X = Line through the superior border of the iliac bone

Y = Line through the sacro-iliac joint

Z = Line through the most inferior part of the sacrum/coccyx

The normal value is considered to be: 0.7–1.0

Figure 1.28a,b Calculation of the sacral ratio.

Lateral Sacral Radiograph

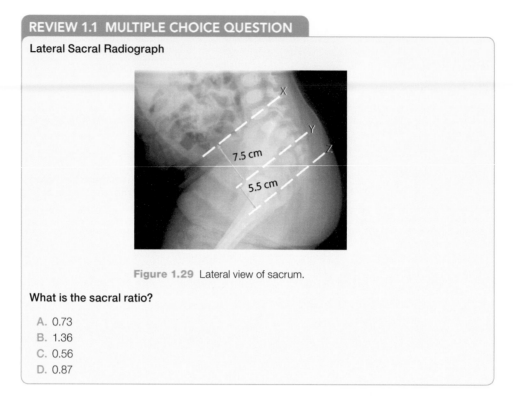

Figure 1.29 Lateral view of sacrum.

What is the sacral ratio?

A. 0.73
B. 1.36
C. 0.56
D. 0.87

ANTERIOR–POSTERIOR (AP) VIEW

In the AP view, it is difficult to draw the lines accurately, and once again the sacrum/coccyx appears to be absent, in this case due to the tilt of the pelvis when the radiograph was taken.

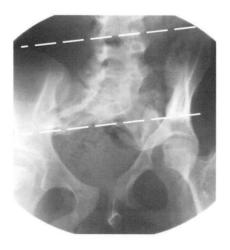

Figure 1.30 AP view.

LATERAL VIEW

In the lateral view shown here the sacrum is short, but the lines to calculate the sacral ratio can be established.

Sacral ratio = 47/76 = 0.62

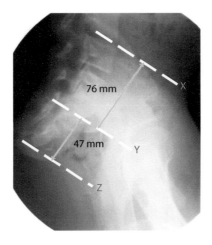

Figure 1.31 Lateral view.

Plain abdominal radiograph of a boy with functional constipation with a cecostomy. No ano-rectal malformation, therefore anticipated normal sacrum.

Sacral ratio = 15/12 = 1.25

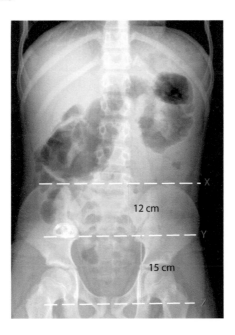

Figure 1.32 AP view.

LEARNING POINTS

- The sacral ratio should be calculated on a *lateral film*.
- AP views of the sacrum can be distorted due to patient positioning, leading to errors in calculation.
- The ratio demonstrates how developed the sacrum is, which correlates with the development of the pelvic muscles and nerves. This information helps to predict continence in patients with an anorectal malformation who have varying degrees of sacral hypodevelopment.

ANSWER

1.1   A

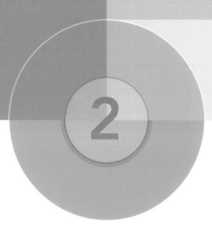

Algorithms for the care of an ARM patient

2

MALE ANORECTAL MALFORMATION

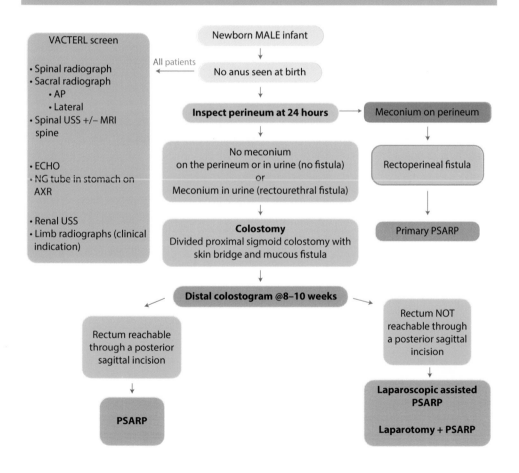

VACTERL screen

- Spinal radiograph
- Sacral radiograph
  - AP
  - Lateral
- Spinal USS +/– MRI spine

- ECHO
- NG tube in stomach on AXR

- Renal USS
- Limb radiographs (clinical indication)

Newborn MALE infant

All patients

No anus seen at birth

Inspect perineum at 24 hours → Meconium on perineum

No meconium on the perineum or in urine (no fistula) or Meconium in urine (rectourethral fistula)

Rectoperineal fistula

Colostomy Divided proximal sigmoid colostomy with skin bridge and mucous fistula

Primary PSARP

Distal colostogram @8–10 weeks

Rectum reachable through a posterior sagittal incision

Rectum NOT reachable through a posterior sagittal incision

PSARP

Laparoscopic assisted PSARP

Laparotomy + PSARP

19

FEMALE ANORECTAL MALFORMATION

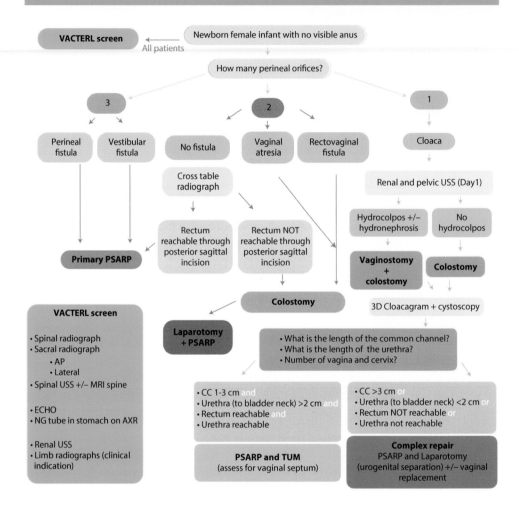

VACTERL screen ← Newborn female infant with no visible anus

All patients

How many perineal orifices?

3

Perineal fistula | Vestibular fistula

2

No fistula | Vaginal atresia | Rectovaginal fistula

1

Cloaca

Cross table radiograph

Rectum reachable through posterior sagittal incision | Rectum NOT reachable through posterior sagittal incision

Primary PSARP

Renal and pelvic USS (Day1)

Hydrocolpos +/− hydronephrosis | No hydrocolpos

Vaginostomy + colostomy | **Colostomy**

Colostomy

3D Cloacagram + cystoscopy

Laparotomy + PSARP

VACTERL screen

• Spinal radiograph
• Sacral radiograph
    • AP
    • Lateral
• Spinal USS +/− MRI spine

• ECHO
• NG tube in stomach on AXR

• Renal USS
• Limb radiographs (clinical indication)

• What is the length of the common channel?
• What is the length of the urethra?
• Number of vagina and cervix?

• CC 1-3 cm and
• Urethra (to bladder neck) >2 cm and
• Rectum reachable and
• Urethra reachable

• CC >3 cm or
• Urethra (to bladder neck) <2 cm or
• Rectum NOT reachable or
• Urethra not reachable

PSARP and TUM
(assess for vaginal septum)

Complex repair
PSARP and Laparotomy (urogenital separation) +/− vaginal replacement

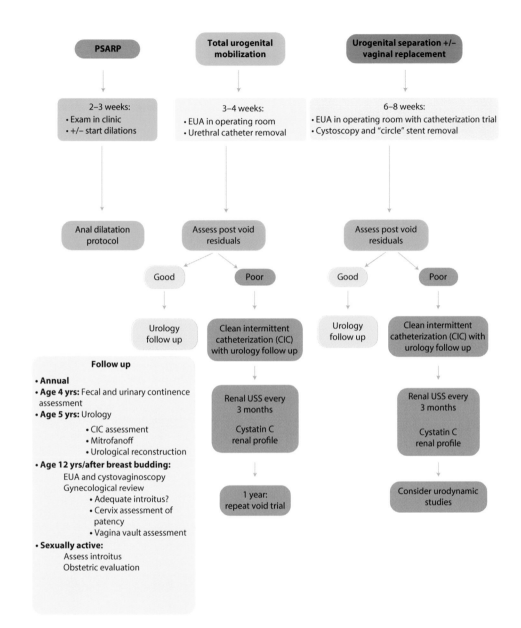

PSARP

Total urogenital mobilization

Urogenital separation +/− vaginal replacement

2–3 weeks:
• Exam in clinic
• +/− start dilations

3–4 weeks:
• EUA in operating room
• Urethral catheter removal

6–8 weeks:
• EUA in operating room with catheterization trial
• Cystoscopy and "circle" stent removal

Anal dilatation protocol

Assess post void residuals

Assess post void residuals

Good

Poor

Good

Poor

Urology follow up

Clean intermittent catheterization (CIC) with urology follow up

Urology follow up

Clean intermittent catheterization (CIC) with urology follow up

Follow up
• **Annual**
• **Age 4 yrs:** Fecal and urinary continence assessment
• **Age 5 yrs:** Urology
   • CIC assessment
   • Mitrofanoff
   • Urological reconstruction
• **Age 12 yrs/after breast budding:**
   EUA and cystovaginoscopy
   Gynecological review
      • Adequate introitus?
      • Cervix assessment of patency
      • Vagina vault assessment
• **Sexually active:**
   Assess introitus
   Obstetric evaluation

Renal USS every 3 months

Cystatin C renal profile

Renal USS every 3 months

Cystatin C renal profile

1 year: repeat void trial

Consider urodynamic studies

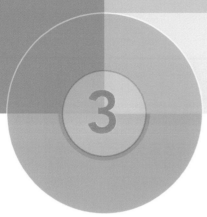

Anorectal malformation newborn: Case study

HISTORY

- You are called to see a newborn male infant (2 hours old) with an anorectal malformation and there is no apparent opening on the perineum.
- On examination, the male infant has a very "flat bottom" with only a minimal gluteal fold.

REVIEW 3.1 MULTIPLE CHOICE QUESTION

What is your management plan for the above case?

A. Wait 24 hours (as in all anorectal malformation patients) to perform a cross table radiograph to establish the position of the rectum.
B. Perform a colostomy within the first 24 hours.
C. Wait for 24 hours and perform the cross table radiograph and then perform a colostomy.
D. Perform an ileostomy within 24 hours.

REVIEW 3.2 MULTIPLE CHOICE QUESTION

You decide to wait 24 hours and perform a cross fire radiograph. What does it show?

A. Perineal fistula
B. Rectoprostatic fistula
C. Bladder neck fistula
D. Rectobulbar fistula
E. High rectum
F. None of the above

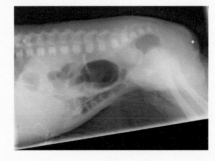

Figure 3.1 Cross-fire image showing rectal air column.

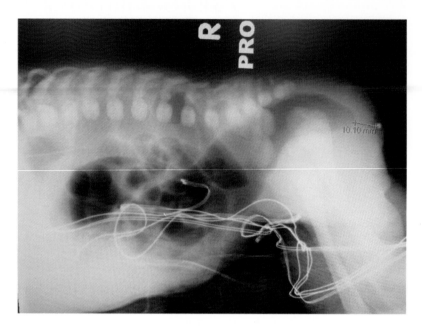

Figure 3.2 Cross fire radiograph. This very different image in another case demonstrates a very low rectum. There was meconium evident of the scrotum and this child could proceed to a primary PSARP.

LEARNING POINTS

- Given the clinical information that you have been provided with (i.e., a very "flat bottom") this child will not likely have a perineal fistula.
- Waiting 24 hours to perform a cross table radiograph before proceeding to a colostomy is best to see if there is a fistula.
- Not all infants with an anorectal malformation require a cross table radiograph. If there is meconium staining the urine, for example, the diagnosis of rectourethral/vesical fistula can already be made and the child would require a divided colostomy.
- The cross table radiograph should not be used to diagnose the position of a rectourethral fistula; instead, a high-pressure distal loop colostogram is needed.
- Performing a transverse colostomy or an ileostomy is a poor choice as these tend to prolapse, and the distal segment is hard to clean out. The long distal segment also makes for a very difficult distal colostogram. You need to perform a divided sigmoid colostomy so that you can perform the distal loop colostogram prior to the definitive repair in order to assess for the presence and hence position of the fistula and the distal rectum.

ANSWERS

3.1   C
3.2   E

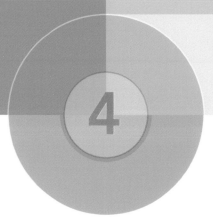

Neonatal colostomy no. 1: Case study

DIVIDED SIGMOID COLOSTOMY WITH MUCOUS FISTULA AND SKIN BRIDGE

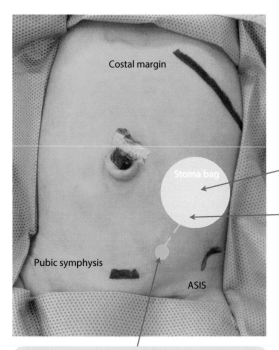

Costal margin

Stoma positioning:
- Far enough away from umbilicus and bony landmarks to enable adhesion of stoma bag and to minimize leakage
- Easy nursing care

Stoma bag

Skin bridge:
- Stoma not placed in the wound
- Minimizes the risk of wound infection

Pubic symphysis

ASIS

Mucous Fistula:
- This child has a rectourethral fistula
- The colostomy and the mucous fistula should be separate so that the mucous fistula is not included in the stoma bag, to minimize spillage of stool into the distal segment.

Figure 4.1 Newborn's abdomen showing anatomic landmarks used to determine colostomy location.

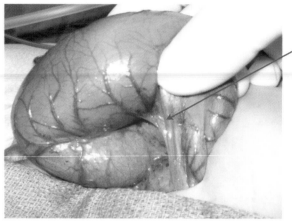

Retroperitoneal attachment:
• **Shown here**

Figure 4.2 Left retroperitoneal attachments.

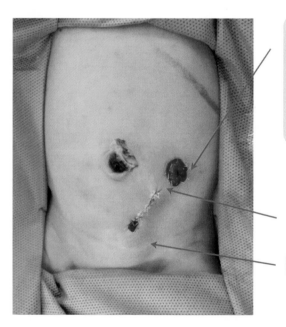

Colostomy:
• The colostomy should be formed at the junction of the descending colon and sigmoid to ensure adequate length remains to perform the posterior sagittal anorectoplasty (PSARP) and bowel pull-through without having to take the colostomy down

Skin bridge

Mucous fistula

Figure 4.3 Colostomy.

LEARNING POINT

▪ The colostomy can also be fashioned laparoscopically, thereby avoiding an incision altogether (Gine et al. 2016).

REFERENCE

Gine C et al. Two-port laparoscopic descending colostomy with separated stomas for anorectal malformations in newborns. *Eur J Pediatr Surg* 2016; 26(5): 462–464.

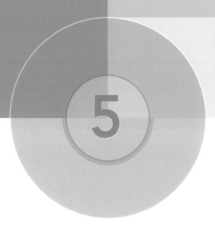

Newborn colostomy no. 2: Case study

5

CASE HISTORY

- This is the case of a newborn infant with an anorectal malformation that was managed initially with a colostomy and mucous fistula.
- The child does not have trisomy 21.

REVIEW 5.1 MULTIPLE CHOICE QUESTION

Considering the distal colostogram below: What is your assessment of the anorectal anomaly?

A. Inadequate colostogram
B. Rectourethral fistula
C. No fistula
D. Perineal fistula

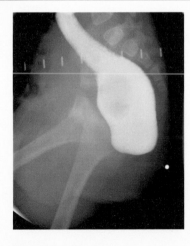

Figure 5.1 Distal colostogram in a male with ARM.

REVIEW 5.2 MULTIPLE CHOICE QUESTION

In a patient with trisomy 21, what is the likelihood of finding this anatomic variation?

A. 5%
B. 25%
C. 5%
D. 95%

ANSWERS

5.1   C
5.2   D

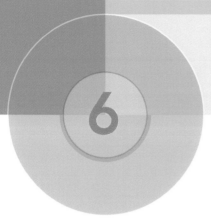

Newborn with ARM and a urologic problem: Case study

6

CASE HISTORY

- This is the plain radiograph of a newborn male infant with an anorectal malformation managed with a divided colostomy.
- **Spine:** He had imaging of his spine as a newborn infant that did not reveal any abnormality or spinal cord tethering.
- **Cardiac:** Echocardiogram was normal.
- **Renal:** Will be discussed in more detail.

What is your interpretation of this radiograph?

The radiograph demonstrates a sacral anomaly, hemi-vertebrae, and scoliosis.

What other investigations does this child require?

The child needs full VACTERL screening investigations.

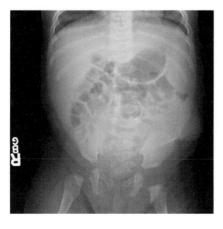

Figure 6.1 Plain abdominal radiograph.

REVIEW 6.1 MULTIPLE CHOICE QUESTION

What does this ultrasound image demonstrate?

A. Right hydronephrosis
B. Left hydronephrosis and thin renal cortex
C. Normal left kidney

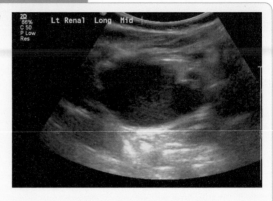

Figure 6.2 Kidney ultrasound image.

What imaging/investigation would you perform now?

A MAG-3 (mercapto acetyl triglycine) is then performed, which demonstrates:

- Poor left renal function
- Split function:
- Left: 7%
- Right: 93%

Discuss how you will manage the renal system?

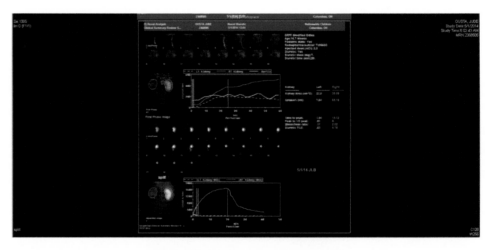

Figure 6.3 Renal scan.

REVIEW 6.2 MULTIPLE CHOICE QUESTION

What is the level of the fistula shown in the distal colostogram below?

A. Rectobulbar fistula
B. Rectoprostatic fistula
C. Bladder neck fistula
D. None of the above

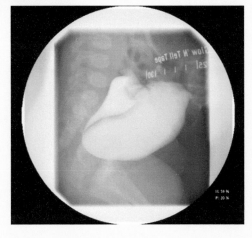

Figure 6.4 Distal colostogram.

LEARNING POINTS

- **Urological:**
  - Initially, this patient required a left ureterostomy in order to decompress the renal system and help prevent urinary tract infection. A future potential use of this dilated ureter is to consider it as tissue for bladder augmentation, if required.
  - The child ultimately underwent a left nephroureterectomy at the time of colostomy closure.
- **Anorectal:**
  - The anorectal malformation is a bladder neck fistula as demonstrated by the distal colostogram.
  - A high rectum such as this is associated with urologic problems as were seen in this case.

ANSWERS

6.1   B
6.2   C

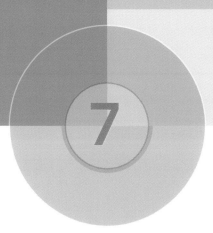

What size does the anus need to be? Anal Hegar sizing: Case study

7

- You are asked to review two newborn infants in the neonatal unit. There are concerns from the neonatologists that the anus is small, and the child has not passed meconium.

REVIEW 7.1 MULTIPLE CHOICE QUESTION

Infant 1: 28-week premature infant weighing 2.26 kg. **What Hegar size should the anus be?**

A. 6
B. 14
C. 10
D. 12

REVIEW 7.2 MULTIPLE CHOICE QUESTION

Infant 2: Term infant weighing 3.8 kg. **What Hegar size should the anus be?**

A. 10
B. 12
C. 16
D. 15

To calculate the Hegar size of the anus in a newborn infant, use the formula below:

Anal diameter in mm (Hegar size) = 7 + (1.3 × weight in kg)

Table 7.1 Newborns

Patient weight (kg)	Mean anal diameter (mm)/Hegar size
1.0–1.5	8.6
1.5–2.0	9.1
2.0–2.5	9.7
2.5–3.0	10.4
3.0–3.5	11.1
3.5–4.0	12.0
4.0–4.5	12.8

Table 7.2 Older child

Patient age	Mean anal diameter (mm)/Hegar size
1–4 months	12
4–8 months	13
8–12 months	14
1–3 years	15
3–12 years	16
>12 years	17

ANSWERS

7.1	C
7.2	B

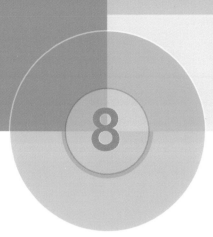

Newborn male with no anal opening and meconium in the urinary stream: Case study

8

CASE HISTORY

- A newborn male infant is having his routine newborn examination.
- The clinical findings of the perineum and anus are shown in the image below.
- There is no opening on the perineum.

REVIEW 8.1 MULTIPLE CHOICE QUESTION

Here you see the image of a male infant. The nurses have reported seeing meconium in the urinary stream.

What type of anorectal malformation are you most likely to see when you perform a distal loop colostogram through the mucous fistula?

A. Perineal fistula
B. Rectobulbar fistula
C. Rectoprostatic fistula
D. Bladder neck fistula
E. No fistula

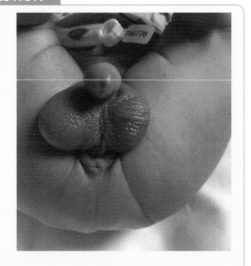

Figure 8.1 Newborn male with no anal opening and meconium in the urine.

Why do you come to this conclusion?

- Flat bottom
- Anal dimple very close to the scrotum

Both of these findings are associated with a high malformation such as a bladder neck fistula.

ANSWER

8.1   D

Newborn who has failed to pass meconium: Case study

9

- This is the case of a newborn male infant (born at full term) with a birth weight of 3.2 kg.
- There was no passage of meconium in the initial 24–48 hours, and this was associated with poor feeding, abdominal distension, and bilious vomiting.

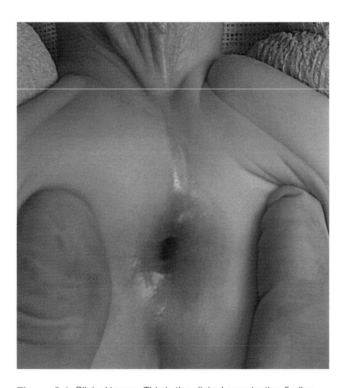

Figure 9.1 Clinical image. This is the clinical examination finding.

REVIEW 9.1 MULTIPLE CHOICE QUESTION

Which of the following would be included in your differential diagnosis based on the information you have been provided with?

A. Hirschsprung disease
B. Rectal atresia
C. Small bowel atresia
D. Malrotation
E. All of the above

REVIEW 9.2 MULTIPLE CHOICE QUESTION

Does this child have a sacral abnormality?

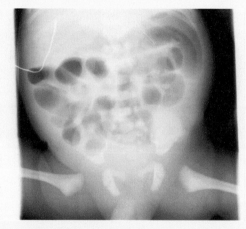

Figure 9.2 Newborn radiograph.

A. Yes
B. No
C. Requires further evaluation with magnetic resonance imaging of the spine/pelvis

REVIEW 9.3 MULTIPLE CHOICE QUESTION

Malrotation has been excluded on an upper gastrointestinal study. This is the plain abdominal radiograph.

What is the most likely diagnosis, given all the information you have been provided with?

A. Hirschsprung disease
B. Rectal atresia
C. Small bowel atresia

REVIEW 9.4 MULTIPLE CHOICE QUESTION

In order to confirm the diagnosis as stated above, what is your next step in the management of this patient?

A. Open a colostomy
B. Perform a contrast enema
C. Attempt to pass 10–12-F catheter into the anus

You attempt to pass a rectal catheter but are unable to advance beyond 3–4 cm. There is no meconium at the tip of the catheter on withdrawal.

REVIEW 9.5 MULTIPLE CHOICE QUESTION

This is a case of rectal atresia. What further investigations need to be performed before the definitive repair?

A. Echocardiogram, renal ultrasound, distal colostogram, passage of a nasogastric tube
B. Echocardiogram, spinal radiographs, magnetic resonance imaging of the spine
C. Echocardiogram, spinal radiographs, ultrasound of the spine ± magnetic resonance imaging of the spine, renal ultrasound
D. Spinal radiographs, ultrasound of the spine ± magnetic resonance imaging of the spine, renal ultrasound, echocardiogram, passage of a nasogastric tube

REVIEW 9.6 MULTIPLE CHOICE QUESTION

The child is becoming increasingly distended.

How are you going to manage this infant?

A. Colostomy with Hartman's pouch
B. Ileostomy
C. Colostomy and mucous fistula
D. Primary repair

REVIEW 9.7 MULTIPLE CHOICE QUESTION

The child fed well postoperatively and was discharged home.

What is your next step in the management of this child?

A. Contrast enema via the anus
B. Colostogram via the colostomy
C. Colostogram via the mucous fistula

REVIEW 9.8 MULTIPLE CHOICE QUESTION

You are considering a posterior sagittal approach. **Is the rectum reachable through a posterior sagittal incision?**

A. Yes

B. No

REVIEW 9.9 MULTIPLE CHOICE QUESTION

Is there a fistula to the urinary tract demonstrated?

A. Yes

B. No

REVIEW 9.10 MULTIPLE CHOICE QUESTION

Is this an adequately performed distal loop colostogram?

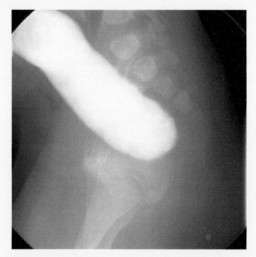

Figure 9.3 Distal colostogram. Distal colostogram through the mucous fistula.

A. Yes

B. No

LEARNING POINTS

- The differential diagnosis of any newborn infant with bilious vomiting should always include malrotation. It is important to exclude this in the first instance with an upper gastrointestinal contrast. An exhaustive list and discussion of the causes of bile-stained emesis can be found in other textbooks.
- This is a case of rectal atresia, which is rare, representing 1% of all anorectal malformations seen. Anal stenosis can have a similar appearance.
- The diagnosis can be missed on the newborn examination because the perineal examination appears normal particularly the anal canal (sometimes the anus appears skin lined, referred to as a funnel anus). Previously, the nursing staff may have reported being unable to insert a rectal thermometer (however, most centers no longer use these) or the radiologists may have failed to instill contrast into the rectum when the diagnosis was suspected.
- The rectum is usually atretic at about 2–4 cm from the anal verge. Anal stenosis can also occur and meconium can be passed, often leading to a diagnosis.
- It is safer to perform a colostomy and mucous fistula in the newborn period so that a distal colostogram can be performed to establish the position of the rectum and the presence of any fistulous communication with the urinary tract.
- The colostogram enables the surgeon to establish whether the rectum is reachable through a posterior sagittal incision if the study is performed correctly and under high pressure, producing a rounded distal rectum as demonstrated in Figure 9.3.
- The infant requires full VACTERL (vertebral, anal, cardiac, tracheo-esophageal, renal, limb) screening, including exclusion of esophageal atresia, renal anomalies, and cardiac defects, with particular attention given to the spine and pre-sacral space, as a pre-sacral mass is seen in ~30% of patients with anal stenesis and rectal atresia.

FURTHER READING

Hamrick M et al. Rectal atresia and stenosis: Unique anorectal malformations. *J Ped Surg* 2012; 47: 1280–1284.

Lane VA, Wood RJ, Reck C, Skerritt C, Levitt M. Rectal atresia and anal stenosis: The difference in the operative technique for these two distinct congenital anorectal malformations. *Tech Coloproctol* 2016; 20(4): 249–254.

ANSWERS

9.1	E
9.2	C
9.3	B
9.4	C
9.5	D
9.6	C
9.7	C
9.8	A
9.9	B
9.10	A

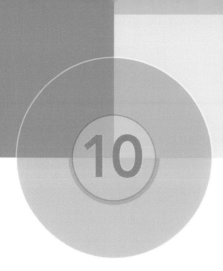
Infant with ARM with a reported no fistula defect—Definitive reconstruction technical details: Case study

CASE HISTORY

- You are asked to see a 2-month-old male infant with an anorectal malformation (ARM).
- You are told by the referring institution that he has an ARM with no fistula. No meconium was seen on the perineum or in the urine by 12 hours of age and he was managed initially with a colostomy and mucous fistula.
- He has trisomy 21.
- His VACTERL screening was negative apart from a small atrial septal defect (ASD) on echocardiogram.

REVIEW 10.1 MULTIPLE CHOICE QUESTION

How are you going to proceed with the management of this child?

A. Primary posterior sagittal anorectoplasty only
B. Primary posterior sagittal anorectoplasty and laparotomy
C. Distal colostogram
D. Pelvic magnetic resonance imaging

REVIEW 10.2 MULTIPLE CHOICE QUESTION

The distal colostogram of this patient is shown below. **What is the diagnosis?**

A. Perineal fistula
B. Rectobulbar fistula
C. No fistula
D. Rectoprostatic fistula

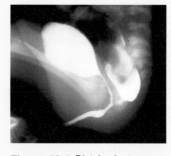

Figure 10.1 Distal colostogram.

LEARNING POINTS

1. If there is meconium on the perineum, it is a perineal fistula, and a primary posterior sagittal anorectoplasty can be performed if the infant is clinically well.
2. If there is no meconium on the perineum *or* there is meconium in the urine, then the patient either has no fistula or a rectourethral fistula, but the position of the fistula is not known at this stage.
   a. The safest procedure for this child is a divided proximal sigmoid colostomy with a mucous fistula.
   b. A distal colostogram should then be performed through the mucous fistula at 8–10 weeks of age.
   c. The distal colostogram gives the surgeon valuable information with regards to the anatomy and this should be used for surgical operative planning.
   d. The distal colostogram enables the surgeon to:
      i. Identify the level of the fistula.
      ii. Establish whether the rectum can be reached through a posterior sagittal incision or whether laparoscopic assistance/laparotomy will be required.
      iii. Establish whether the rectum narrowly tapers at the end or is wide at the distal extent.

The distal colostogram must be assessed on an individual patient basis.

1. Knowing the level of the fistula enables the surgeon to predict where it will be identified intra-operatively, rather than searching blindly and risking damage to the urethra, bladder neck, seminal vesicles, or the vas deferens.
2. The rectum may be low in one patient with a rectoprostatic fistula, but relatively high in another and not reachable through a posterior sagittal incision. So it is not only the location of the fistula that matters, but also the characteristics of the distal rectum.
3. Sacral hypoplasia/agenesis may enable easier access to the rectum through a posterior sagittal incision, so the sacral anatomy should also be assessed. Of course, this also means poor prognosis for bowel control.
4. Bladder neck fistula/rectovesical fistula, as a general rule, require laparoscopic assistance/laparotomy.

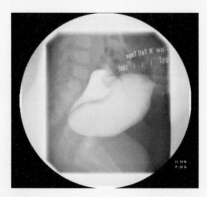

Figure 10.2 Bladder neck fistula. The rectum will not be reached through a posterior sagittal incision and will require transabdominal mobilization, ideally laparoscopically.

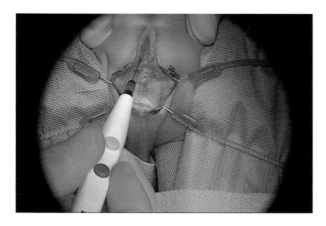

Figure 10.3 Primary posterior sagittal anorectoplasty in a male; operative images for rectobulbar fistula.

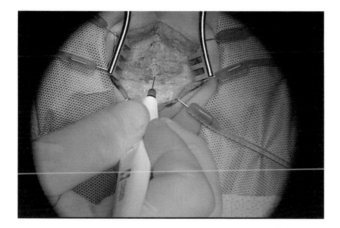

Figure 10.4 Midline dissection ensuring equal distribution of muscle fibers on the left and the right.

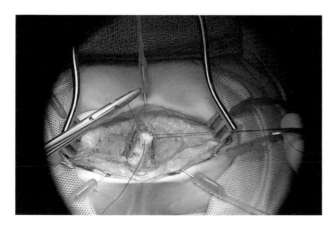

Figure 10.5 Rectum is identified and stay silk sutures are placed.

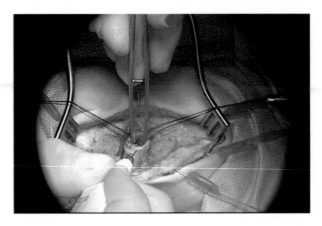

Figure 10.6 Rectum is opened above the position of the fistula, and is opened further until the fistula is seen. This is marked with a silk stay suture.

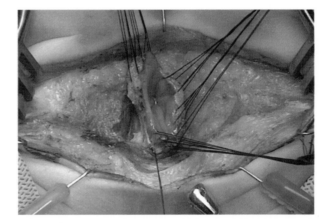

Figure 10.7 The rectum is mobilized off the urethra. The urethra is catheterized.

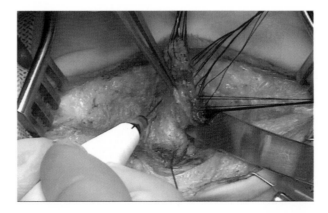

Figure 10.8 In order to find the dissection plane, it is safer and easier to start on the lateral walls of the rectum and then follow the plane anteriorly and dissect off the urethra.

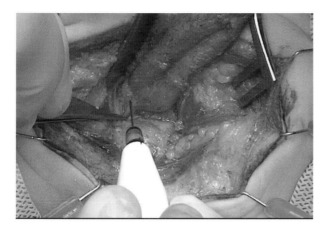

Figure 10.9 Ensure that the dissection is on the wall of the rectum.

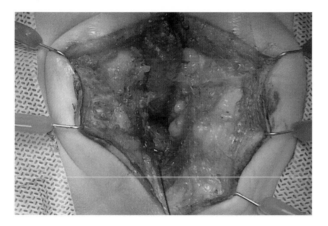

Figure 10.10 The muscle complex is demonstrated here.

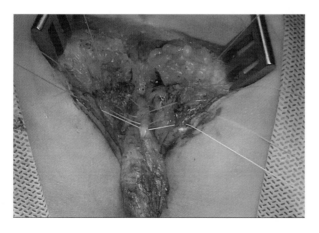

Figure 10.11 The rectum is tacked during the closure of the posterior sagittal incision to prevent future rectal prolapse.

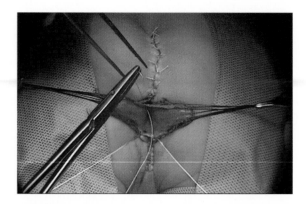

Figure 10.12 The anoplasty is performed using a standard 16-suture technique.

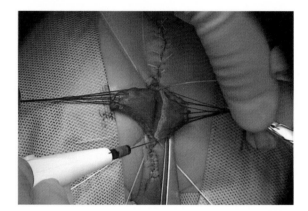

Figure 10.13 The rectum is trimmed.

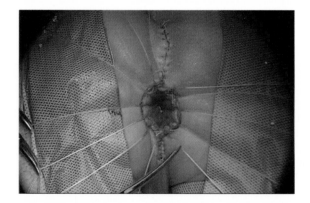

Figure 10.14 The anoplasty is complete.

ANSWERS

10.1   C
10.2   B

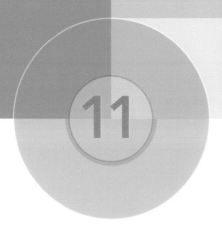

Male anorectal malformation: Case study

11

CASE HISTORY

- This is a newborn male infant with an anorectal malformation seen at 26 hours of age.
- He has undergone his routine VACTERL screening as per the protocol.
- His clinical images are shown below.
- What do you notice on clinical examination?

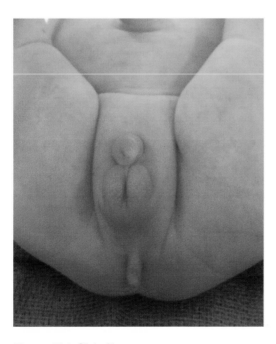

Figure 11.1 Clinical images.

REVIEW 11.1 MULTIPLE CHOICE QUESTION

How are you going to manage this child in the newborn period?

A. Ileostomy
B. Loop colostomy
C. End colostomy
D. Colostomy and mucous fistula

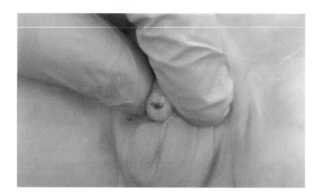

Figure 11.2 Tip of phallus with meconium visible.

LEARNING POINTS

Figure 11.1

Male infant with an anorectal malformation with an associated skin tag in the anal area. The scrotum is abnormal. Both testes are descended.

Figure 11.2

Meconium at the urethral meatus was noted, demonstrating a communication with the urinary tract.

LEARNING POINTS

- In this patient there is a rectourethral fistula and the colon needs to be separated from the urinary tract.
- The raised area (skin tag) marks the center of the sphincter complex and the anoplasty should be centered here.
- It is somewhat anterior, and close to the scrotum, typical of a bladder neck or prostatic fistula.
- A mucous fistula is required to perform the distal colostogram in order to identify the level of the site of the fistula (e.g., rectobulbar or rectoprostatic).
- A loop colostomy should be avoided because fecal material can *potentially* spill into the mucous fistula.

ANSWER

11.1   D

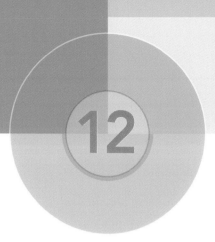

Distal colostogram showing a very short distal segment: Case study

12

CASE HISTORY

- A 2-month-old male infant with an anorectal malformation was diverted at birth with a colostomy and mucous fistula.
- The distal loop colostogram is shown below.

REVIEW 12.1 MULTIPLE CHOICE QUESTION

Is this an adequate colostogram/study?

A. Yes

B. No

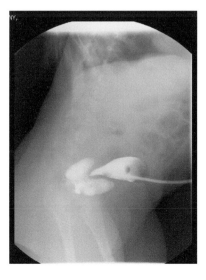

Figure 12.1 Distal colostogram.

REVIEW 12.2 MULTIPLE CHOICE QUESTION

Consider the images in Figure 12.2. **What do you notice?**

    A. No fistula is seen to enter the urethra.
    B. The mucous fistula is too short to reach the perineum.
    C. The rectum is not reachable through a posterior sagittal incision.
    D. All of the above.

REVIEW 12.3 MULTIPLE CHOICE QUESTION

What is the diagnosis?

    A. Rectobladder fistula
    B. Perineal fistula
    C. No fistula
    D. Unable to determine from this study

REVIEW 12.4 MULTIPLE CHOICE QUESTION

How would you approach the definitive repair?

    A. Via the abdomen, mobilize the colostomy and pull through and resect the mucous fistula.
    B. Via the abdomen, mobilize and pull through the mucous fistula, leaving the colostomy untouched and the distal rectum as a Hartmann pouch.
    C. Via the posterior sagittal incision, mobilize the distal rectum only (primary posterior sagittal anorectoplasty only).
    D. Close the stoma, dissect the fistula from the bladder, pull through the newly anastomosed bowel, and fashion a colostomy more proximally.
    E. Answers A or D.
    F. Answers A, B, or D.

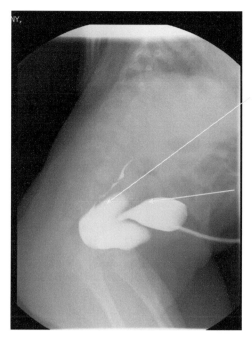

- The distal loop colostogram is an adequate study and the fistula is seen to enter the bladder.

- The mucous fistula is extremely short, and this will be too short to pull-through to the perineum.

- The rectum will not be reachable through a posterior sagittal incision, and this child will require an abdominal approach to divide the fistula from the bladder.

Figure 12.2 Distal colostogram.

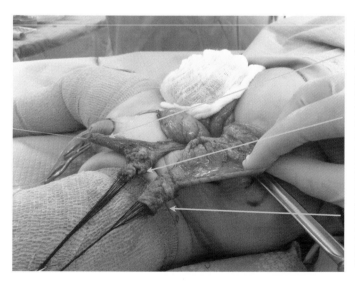

- The fistula has been dissected off the back of the bladder

- Original mucous fistula

- Mobilized colostomy

Figure 12.3 Operative view showing a very short distal segment.

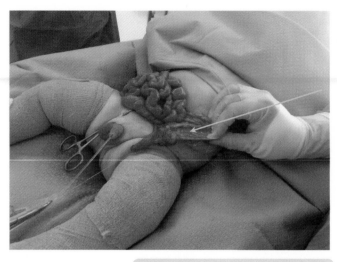

- The mucous fistula and the colostomy have been anastomosed

- This segment will now be pulled through to the perineum

- The patient's native rectum has therefore been preserved which is important

- This will function as a rectal reservoir and improve the chance of continence

A more proximal colostomy is then opened

Figure 12.4 Operative view showing anastomosis of distal segment to proximal colostomy.

LEARNING POINTS

- If possible, it would be best to preserve the mucous fistula for the rectum (**Answer D, Review Question 12.4**). This would, however, require mobilization of the colostomy, re-anastomosis, pull-through of this re-anastomosed segment, and formation of a new (more proximal) ostomy.
- The other option (**Answer A, Review 12.4**), however, would lead to loss of the distal rectum, which is currently inserting into the bladder.
- In this scenario (**Figure 12.2**), both of the above options A and D are reasonable approaches.
    - However, option D is the best option because:
        - The rectal reservoir is retained.
        - With the rectal reservoir *in situ*, hypermotility and fecal incontinence are less likely.
- In this case, there was no real loop to the sigmoid noted when the colostomy was fashioned in the immediate newborn period. Ideally, the surgeon should have recognized this anatomical finding and fashioned the stoma more proximally (e.g., descending colon or even transverse colon, even though this is not the usual approach that is taught) in order to avoid the extremely short mucous fistula, which cannot be utilized for the pull-through without an additional procedure.

ANSWERS

12.1   A
12.2   D
12.3   A
12.4   E

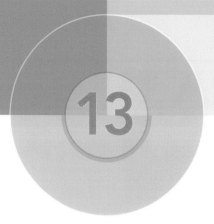

Newborn with an anorectal malformation: Case study

13

- This is a case of a male infant with an anorectal malformation. Consider the questions below.

REVIEW 13.1 MULTIPLE CHOICE QUESTION

What type of anorectal malformation is shown here?

A. Rectobulbar fistula
B. Rectoprostatic fistula
C. Bladder neck fistula

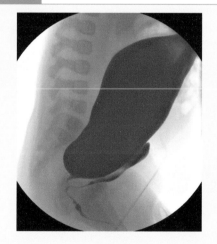

Figure 13.1 Distal colostogram.

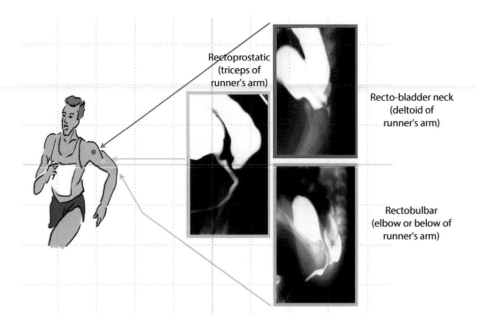

Rectoprostatic
(triceps of
runner's arm)

Recto-bladder neck
(deltoid of
runner's arm)

Rectobulbar
(elbow or below of
runner's arm)

REVIEW 13.2 MULTIPLE CHOICE QUESTION

How would you perform the definitive repair on this patient?

A. Posterior sagittal incision only (primary posterior sagittal anorectoplasty)
B. Laparoscopic-assisted primary posterior sagittal anorectoplasty
C. Laparotomy and primary posterior sagittal anorectoplasty
D. A or B

LEARNING POINTS

- This case illustrates well the borderline between a posterior sagittal and a laparoscopic approach. Both options are reasonable.
- The rectum is high but could be safely reached through a posterior sagittal incision alone, but the surgeon must recognize that it will be difficult and a long rectal dissection will be required. The urinary tract is at risk of injury. The rectum will be found high, above the level of coccyx.
- The rectum is very dilated and likely to make the laparoscopic approach difficult, but this would be a reasonable approach.

ANSWERS

13.1   A
13.2   D

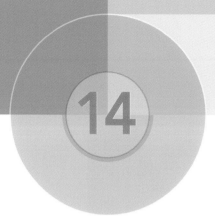

Four-month-old with difficulty stooling: Case study

14

CASE HISTORY

- This is a 4-month-old boy who presented to the clinic. The parent expressed concerns that the child was having difficulty stooling.
- On examination, the anal opening appears to be narrow. You pass a Hegar dilator #8 and it is snug. Then you organize a contrast enema as shown below.

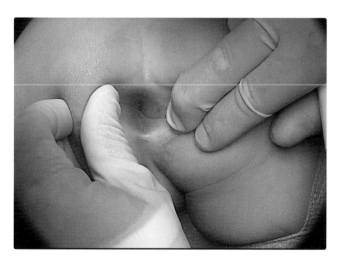

Figure 14.1 Clinical image showing a normal location of an anal opening that appears narrow, and skin-lined, consistent with anal stenosis.

What further imaging is required before this child has the definitive repair?

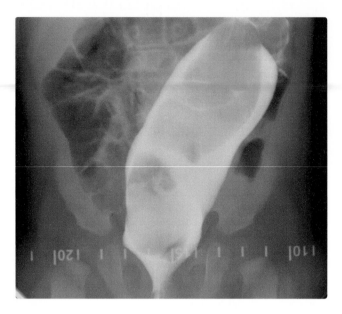

Figure 14.2 Contrast enema showing a very dilated rectosigmoid.

LEARNING POINTS

- This child has anal stenosis.
- There is a known association with a pre-sacral mass in this malformation and the child therefore needs a magnetic resonance imaging scan before the definitive repair.
  - If a pre-sacral mass is present, this can be resected at the same time.
- If such a mass is detected it is likely a teratoma. A meningocele is also possible, and if the mass has any connection to the dura, neurosurgery will need to get involved.
- Full VACTERL screening would also be indicated in this case.

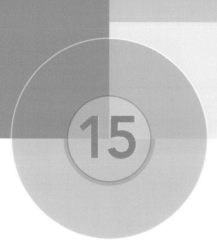

15

Three-month-old female with a possible anorectal malformation: Case study

CASES

- Below are two clinical images of the female perineum.
- In both cases (A and B) the urethra and the vagina appear normal on examination.

REVIEW 15.1 MULTIPLE CHOICE QUESTION

Clinical Image A: This is the clinical image of a female perineum. The urethra and the vagina are normal.

What is the diagnosis?

A. Normal anus, but anteriorly located
B. Normal anatomy
C. Perineal fistula
D. Vestibular fistula

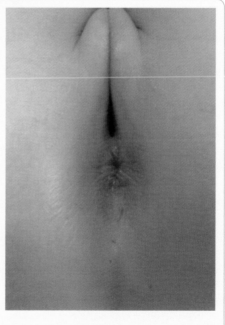

Figure 15.1 Female perineum referred for a possible anorectal malformation.

REVIEW 15.2 MULTIPLE CHOICE QUESTION

Clinical Image B: This is the clinical image of a female perineum. The urethra and the vagina are normal.

What is the diagnosis?

A. Normal anatomy
B. Normal anus, but anteriorly located
C. Perineal fistula
D. Vestibular fistula

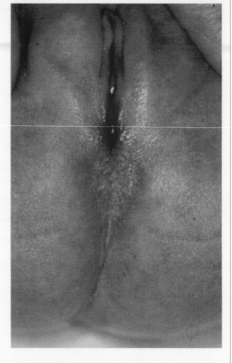

Figure 15.2 Female perineum referred for a possible anorectal malformation.

LEARNING POINTS

To assess the anus, you need to establish:

1. Is the anus within the sphincter complex?
2. Is the perineal body an adequate size?
3. Is the anus of a normal size when calibrated?

Clinical Figure 15.1 shows

- An anterior ectopic anus and calibrates to the size of a normal anus.
- The anus is within the sphincter complex and the perineal body will increase with age.
- No surgery is required.

Clinical Figure 15.2 shows

- A perineal fistula, an opening that is too small.
- The opening is anterior to the sphincter complex and the perineal body is too short.
- Surgery is required.

CASE HISTORY

- You are asked to review a newborn female infant with a suspected anorectal malformation.
- Your clinical findings are shown in the image below.
- A size 12 Hegar passes without difficulty.
- Congenital malformation characterized by a wet sulcus extending from the posterior fourchette to the anterior edge of the anus.

REVIEW 15.3 MULTIPLE CHOICE QUESTION

Is the anal opening well centered within the sphincter complex?

A. Yes
B. No
C. Unable to tell

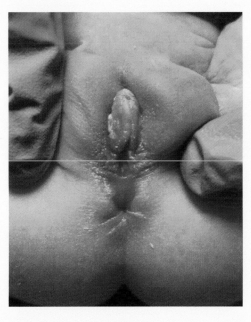

Figure 15.3 Image of perineum.

REVIEW 15.4 MULTIPLE CHOICE QUESTION

What is your diagnosis?

A. Anterior anus
B. Perineal fistula
C. Perineal groove
D. Rectovestibular fistula

LEARNING POINTS

- This is a rare condition.
- The perineal body appears to be red and inflamed. This is a perineal groove and is a relatively common finding.
- On occasion, this is mucosal, but tends to resolve spontaneously and does not require surgical excision. Usually, by the age of 1 year, it becomes epithelialized.
- Provided the anal opening is within the sphincter and is of adequate size, the surgical intervention is required
- Surgical excision has been reported for cosmetic reasons and due to persistent production of mucous.

FURTHER READING

Mullassery D et al. Perineal groove. *J Ped Surg* 2006, 42, E41–E43.

ANSWERS

15.1	A
15.2	C
15.3	A
15.4	C

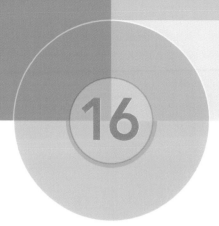

H-type rectovaginal fistula: Case study

16

CASE HISTORY

- A 6-year-old female comes to your clinic with her parents. The parents are concerned that she is stooling from her vagina. She has been stooling normally but stains her underwear, especially when she has loose stools and mom thinks the stain is near her vaginal area. Previous clinicians have told the parents that the anatomy is normal and that stool in the vagina is due to poor wiping. There is no previous history of colorectal surgery. You suspect that she may have a rectovaginal fistula.

QUESTIONS

1. What additional information would you like from the parents?
2. Where are rectovaginal fistulae typically located? Are they congenital or acquired?
3. What associated rectal abnormality can be seen with H-type fistulae?
4. What additional workup is required in the preoperative assessment of this patient?

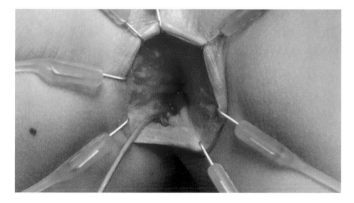

Figure 16.1 Rectovaginal fistula. Note the lacrimal duct probe in a crypt which passes into the vagina. The patient is prone. Findings at examination under anesthesia demonstrate a rectovaginal fistula.

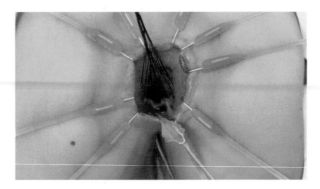

Figure 16.2 Operative images. The patient is PRONE. For the repair of this H-type rectovaginal fistula, the dentate line has been hidden by the retracting pins and 1 cm above the dentate line has been marked with ink. The fistula is demonstrated by the lacrimal duct probe. Silk stay sutures have been placed.

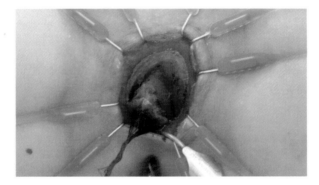

Figure 16.3 Trans-anal circumferential dissection is then performed in the Swenson plane.

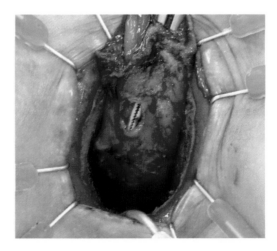

Figure 16.4 Trans-anal dissection is performed and the rectum has been mobilized for 6–8 cm. The fistula is demonstrated with the dissecting forceps in the rectum.

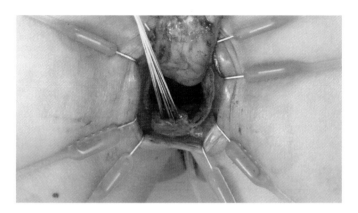

Figure 16.5 The fistulous opening into the vagina is shown here. Sutures have been placed circumferentially around the fistula, the tract is excised, and the vagina repaired.

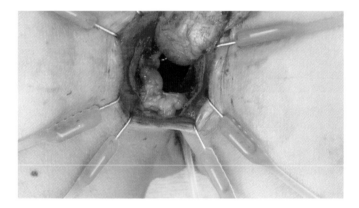

Figure 16.6 An incision is made in parallel with the muscle fibers on the left-hand side. Ischiorectal fat is mobilized and sutured to cover the site of the fistula (Levitt et al. 2014.)

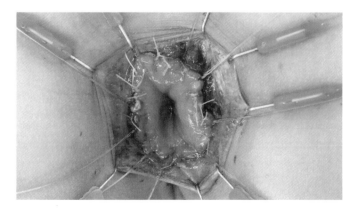

Figure 16.7 The anoplasty is completed in the standard fashion.

LEARNING POINTS

■ Rectovaginal fistulae can present as labial abscesses or perirectal abscesses and the surgeon should ask about previous episodes of perineal sepsis. The child may also have a history of constipation and recurrent urinary tract infection (Lawal et al. 2011).

■ Rectovaginal fistulae are known to be associated with rectal stenosis and a history of constipation, and this should be examined for. Patients with a H-type rectovaginal fistulae may have rectal stenosis, and this is known to be associated with a pre-sacral mass; therefore, the child should undergo a spinal magnetic resonance imaging scan.

■ H-type rectovaginal fistulae are rare in the U.S. population, representing only 0.7% of all anorectal malformations. The incidence is much higher in the Asian population. Many these cases might be acquired rather than congenital.

■ All patients with a perianal or labial abscess should have a rectal examination in order to rule out anal stenosis.

Location of the fistulae

■ **Congenital**: Fistula is found in the midline extending from the dentate line (anal crypt) to the vestibule. Sigmoidoscopy and contrast studies can easily miss this abnormality and often only careful inspection in this location will identify the fistula.

■ **Acquired**: Fistula is off the midline and most likely associated with a previous perirectal abscess.

REFERENCES

Lawal et al. Management of H type rectovestibular and rectovaginal fistulas. *J Ped Surg* 2011, 46, 1226–1230.

Levitt et al. The Gonzalez hernia revisited: Use of the ischiorectal fat pad to aid in the repair of rectovaginal and rectourethral fistulae. *J Ped Surg* 2014, 49(8), 1308–1310.

17

Female ARM preoperative and operative management: Case study

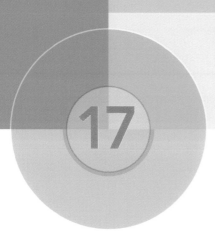

CASE HISTORY

A 10-month-old female infant with an anorectal malformation is referred. She has been managed with a divided sigmoid colostomy and mucous fistula.

REVIEW 17.1 MULTIPLE CHOICE QUESTION

This is a female infant with what type of anorectal malformation?

A. Perineal fistula
B. Rectovestibular fistula
C. Cloaca
D. Rectovaginal fistula

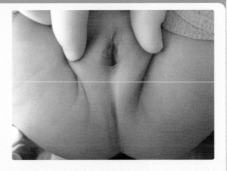

Figure 17.1 Perineum of a newborn female.

PREOPERATIVE PLANNING

What initial investigations does this child require?

1. Newborn: Pelvic ultrasound to assess for hydrocolpos
2. Newborn: VACTERL screening: renal USS, spinal USS, X-ray of the spine and sacrum, echocardiogram
3. First 2–3 months of life (non-urgent) examination under anesthesia (EUA)/cysto-vaginoscopy and cloacagram to assess:
   a. Length of the common channel
   b. Length of the urethra to the bladder neck (from the urethral take-off)
   c. Presence of a vaginal septum and vaginal anatomy
   d. Location of the distal rectum

RESULTS IN THIS CASE

RENAL

- Normal kidneys
- No hydronephrosis

PELVIC USS

- Double vagina with uterine didelphys
- No hydrocolpos

SPINAL ULTRASOUND

- Normal spine, no tethered cord
- Tip of the conus at L2

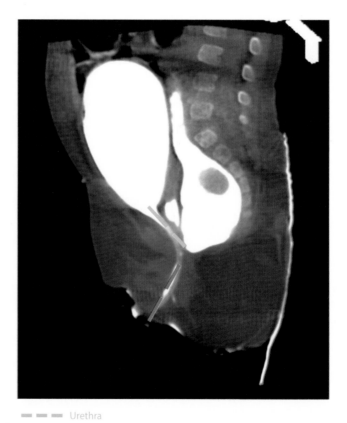

— — — Urethra

━ ━ ━ Common Channel

Figure 17.2 Cloacagram. The urethra, vagina, and rectum are demonstrated to enter into the common channel.

SACRAL RADIOGRAPHS

- Sacral ratio 0.76
- No hemisacrum

ECHO

- Normal

LIMBS

- No abnormalities

With this information, the surgeons need to establish the operative management plan.

The options for the repair are:

- Total urogenital mobilization (TUM).
- Leave the common channel as the urethra and separate the vagina from the common channel.
- Vaginal replacement if necessary.

INTRA-OPERATIVE DECISIONS

There are important pieces of information that need to be established from the preoperative investigations that will assist the surgeon in planning the definitive operative repair.

1. What is the length of the common channel?
   - The length of the common channel is the most important piece of information required in order to best plan for the repair. If the length of the common channel is <3 cm, then the repair is less complex and the anatomy is more predictable and a total urogenital mobilization is likely possible, however, once the common channel is >3 cm in length, the operative repair is more complex and technically demanding.
   - When the common channel is at the intermediate range of 3–4 cm in length, the decision making can be more complicated and there are important additional factors to take into account, as detailed below.
2. What is the length of the urethra? What is the length of the urethra from the common channel/"urethral take-off" to the bladder neck?
   - The length of the urethra is another important length to establish on cystoscopy. The 3D cloacagram is an extremely valuable investigation as well, as the anatomy is clearly defined, and the measurements of the common channel length and urethral length are likely to be more accurate than relying on the cystoscopy alone.
   - The reason for measuring this length (in addition to the common channel length) is to aid in the decision-making process with regards to the technique used for the operative repair.
   - If a TUM is performed, then the bladder neck and the vagina are mobilized en bloc to reach the perineum.

- If the urethral length is very short (<1.5 cm), then after a TUM procedure, the bladder neck would end up being very close to the perineum, and the child is likely to have bladder neck incompetence and persistent urinary leakage. Therefore, a TUM should be avoided.
- If the urethral length is >1.5 cm, then it is appropriate to perform a TUM, as the ultimate position of the bladder neck will be more than 1.5 cm from the perineum.

3. What is the distance of the vagina to the perineum? Is there a vaginal septum that requires resection?
- The next measurement to establish, before committing to the TUM intra-operatively, is whether the vagina will reach the perineum with a TUM.
- Previously, the TUM has been advocated. Initially, the TUM is started from the perineum, and when there is inadequate length, the TUM is continued from a transabdominal approach.
- After the TUM has been approached from both the perineum and the abdomen, and the urethra and vagina are still too short to reach the perineum, there are difficult decisions to be made and an increased risk of complications.
- Aborting the TUM at this stage and then making the decision to separate the vagina and the urethra is problematic, because now dissections on both the anterior and posterior urethra have been done, which can compromise its blood supply. Sometimes, though, mobilizing the TUM up into the abdomen allows the surgeon to gain enough length for it to reach.
- When the decision is made from the outset to separate the vagina and urethra, the anterior wall of the common channel is left untouched, minimizing the risk of disruption to the blood supply.

CONCLUSION

We would therefore advocate the following approach:

- **For <3 cm common channel:** TUM, provided the urethral length is at least 1.5 cm.
- **For >3 cm common channel and with a short urethral length:** the common channel becomes the urethra with dissection of the vagina(s) off of the posterior aspect of the common channel with vaginal replacement (as required).

If there is doubt about the feasibility of mobilizing the urethra and the vagina to the perineum, we would suggest that the surgeon elects to preserve the common channel as the urethra and minimizes disruption to its blood supply from the outset.

DEFINITIVE RECONSTRUCTION

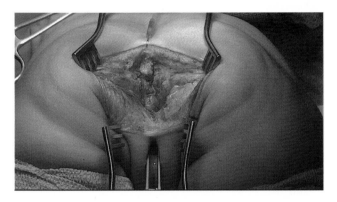

Figure 17.3 Total urogenital mobilization. Posterior sagittal incision, with exposure of the rectum.

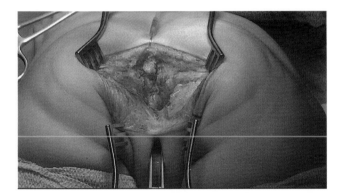

Figure 17.4 The rectum is being opened here. Opening the rectum moving anteriorly will lead to the common channel distally.

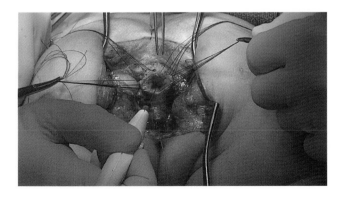

Figure 17.5 The vagina has been opened and the rectum has been fully mobilized.

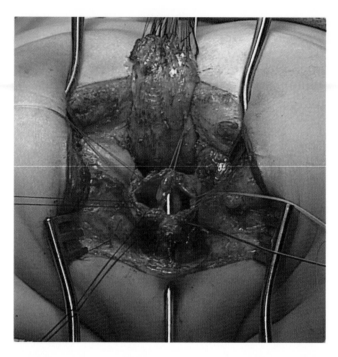

Figure 17.6 The common channel is being laid open with cautery, with cutting on top of the Hegar dilator.

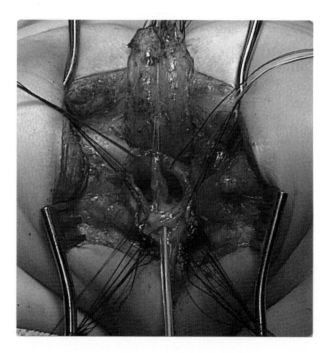

Figure 17.7 The common channel has been laid open (~2 cm). A vaginal septum is clearly demonstrated. The urethra is visible and a urinary catheter has been placed.

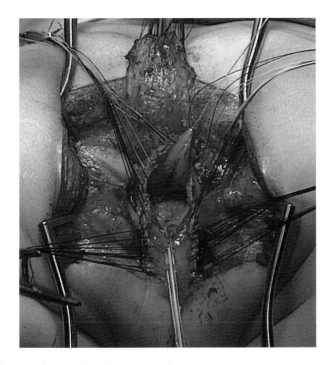

Figure 17.8 The vaginal septum has been resected.

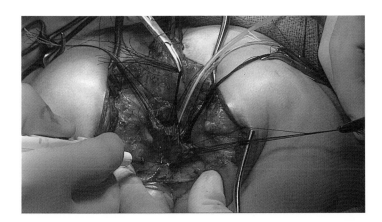

Figure 17.9 Total urogenital mobilization. The anterior wall of the common channel is being dissected.

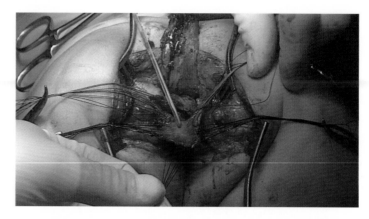

Figure 17.10 Total urogenital mobilization. The urethra and vagina have been mobilized so that these structures reach the perineum.

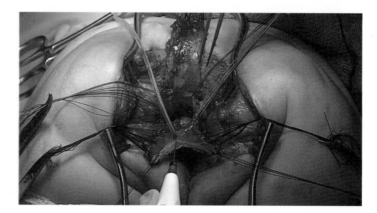

Figure 17.11 The common channel is being split back to the urethral orifice. The excess common channel tissue will be used to fashion the labia.

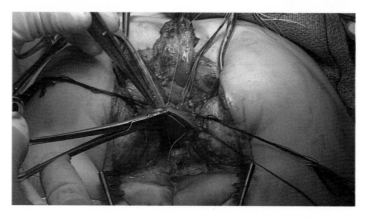

Figure 17.12 The mobilized structures are being sutured to the perineum.

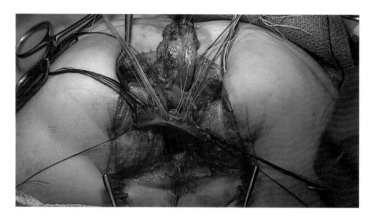

Figure 17.13 Sutures are placed.

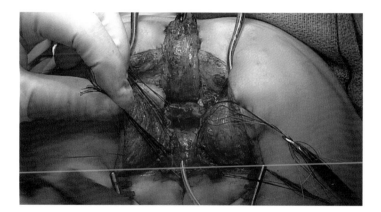

Figure 17.14 Sutures are tied and the urethral orifice is seen to be at the level of the skin.

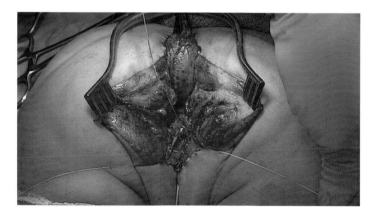

Figure 17.15 The vaginal orifice is established on the perineum.

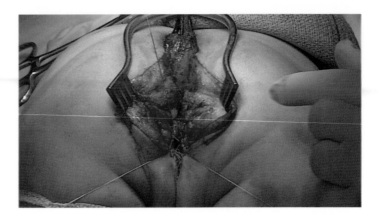

Figure 17.16 The vaginal introitus is created.

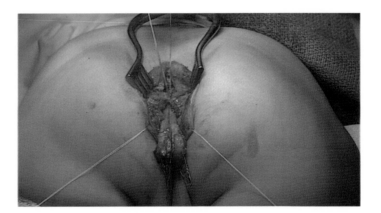

Figure 17.17 The rectum is positioned within the sphincter complex.

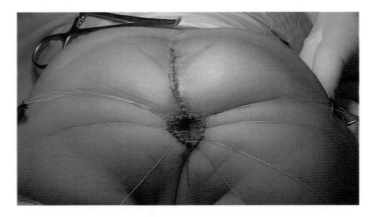

Figure 17.18 Postoperative image.

LEARNING POINTS

1. A cystoscopy and cloacagram are recommended in order to establish the length of the common channel, the length of the urethra (from the common channel to the bladder neck), and the distance the vagina needs to be mobilized to the perineum.
2. If there is doubt about the feasibility of mobilizing the urethra and the vagina to the perineum, we would suggest that the surgeon elects to preserve the common channel as the urethra and minimizes disruption to its blood supply from the outset.

ANSWER

17.1   C

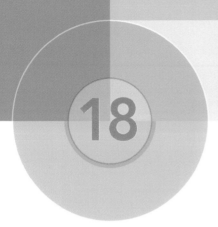

Neonatal evaluation of a child with ARM: Case study

18

CASE HISTORY

- A 36-week gestation newborn female infant is being cared for in the neonatal unit.
- The infant is distended and the nursing staff report frothing/bubbles coming from the mouth.
- This is the plain abdominal radiograph taken just after birth.

MANAGEMENT

- How are you going to proceed with the management of this infant?
- What do you expect to find on general examination?
- What are your main concerns?
- Are there any other investigations you would like in the first 24 hours?

Consider the multiple choice questions below.

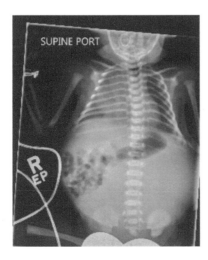

Figure 18.1 Plain radiograph. What is your interpretation of this radiograph?

REVIEW 18.1 MULTIPLE CHOICE QUESTION

Is there an associated tracheoesophageal fistula (TEF)?

A. Yes
B. No
C. Unable to tell from the radiograph

REVIEW 18.2 MULTIPLE CHOICE QUESTION

This child potentially has VACTERL association. What else do you need to exclude in this child as part of the VACTERL screen?

A. Ventricular septal defect/atrial septal defect (VSD/ASD), limb anomalies, renal anomalies, spinal anomalies
B. Limb anomalies, cardiac anomalies, choanal atresia
C. Renal anomalies, spinal anomalies

REVIEW 18.3 MULTIPLE CHOICE QUESTION

The child has an anorectal malformation on clinical examination and a doughy abdominal wall. The child has not passed urine. The radiograph demonstrates a large opacity within the abdomen. **What is this likely to represent?**

A. Wilms' tumor
B. Ascites
C. Distended bladder
D. Distended vagina
E. Distended colon

Why was the abdomen distended in utero?
Likely this was due to urinary ascites, with egress of urine into the peritoneal space via the fallopian tubes.

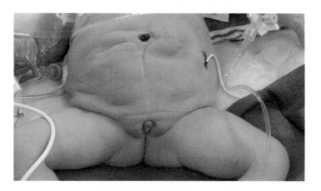

Figure 18.2 Clinical image.

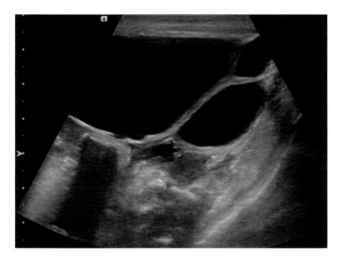

Figure 18.3 Renal/abdominal USS. This is a single image from the renal USS, showing a "large oval cystic structure" on the left side of the abdomen, with a septum. The left kidney is moderately hydronephrotic with a dilated and tortuous ureter and the right kidney is also hydronephrotic. There are concerns that the kidneys are obstructed bilaterally.

REVIEW 18.4 MULTIPLE CHOICE QUESTION

How are you going to manage the obstructed kidneys?

A. Bilateral nephrostomies

B. Bladder catheter and repeat the renal ultrasound in 12 hours

C. Drain the hydrocolpos with a vaginostomy

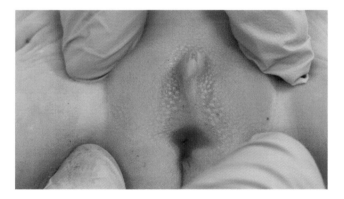

Figure 18.4 Perineum. Closer inspection of the perineum. The infant has been stooling through this single perineal opening which is more posterior than the normal opening of a cloaca and raises suspicion for a posterior cloacal variant. Urine is also draining via this opening.

LEARNING POINTS AND EXPLANATION

1. The radiograph reveals several abnormalities:
   a. Esophageal atresia with a distal TEF.
   b. Sacral anomaly.
   c. Large fluid-filled mass in the abdomen, which is likely to represent a hydrocolpos.
2. On examination, therefore, one would expect to find VACTERL-associated anomalies.
   a. Anorectal malformation cloacal anomaly given suspicion of hydrocolpos on the radiograph.
   b. Heart murmur/cardiac lesion.
   c. Limb anomalies.
3. Main concerns for this child in the first few hours of life are:
   a. Airway, breathing, and circulation.
   b. If the infant is intubated, the TEF is a significant concern due to the potential risk of increasing abdominal distention (air passing through the fistula into the gastrointestinal tract) leading to distension of the stomach, splinting of the diaphragm, and respiratory compromise.
   c. The hydrocolpos is likely to be causing obstruction to the upper renal tracts and requires decompression as a matter of urgency. The large oval cystic structure with a septum on the renal USS represents a distended hemivagina with a septum. This septum needs to be divided in order for both sides to drain.
   d. Does the child need a colostomy?
4. Anesthetic review: echocardiogram.
5. Assessment of the spine is required by spinal ultrasound, but this is not urgent.

SUGGESTED MANAGEMENT PLAN

1. Ligation of the TEF as a matter of urgency ± esophageal atresia repair.
2. Vaginostomy with division of the vaginal septum as demonstrated on pelvic USS.
3. Formation of a divided colostomy.
4. Careful observation of hydronephrosis following hydrocolpos drainage (hydronephrosis should resolve slowly over 1–2 weeks).
5. Definitive surgical repair once thriving (at least 6 months).

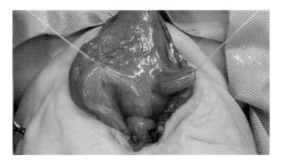

Figure 18.5 Bilateral hydrocolpos. This child has a cloacal anomaly and the fluid-filled cystic structure on the renal USS is a distended vagina (hydrocolpos) as demonstrated in this clinical image. The distended vagina has been delivered through the midline laparotomy incision.

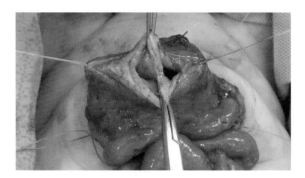

Figure 18.6 Vaginal septum exposed via an incision in the dome of the vagina.

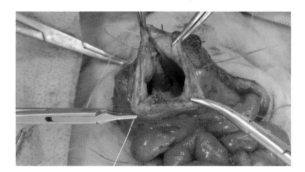

Figure 18.7 Excised vaginal septum.

- The vagina has been opened and the vaginal septum is identified.
- The vaginal septum needs to be divided in order for both halves of the structure to drain adequately. This is done transabdominally, and then a single tube can drain both sides of the hydrocolpos.

The distended vagina causes compression of the ureters as they enter the bladder, leading to the bilateral hydronephrosis seen on the renal USS.

- The vaginal septum has been divided.

The right ureter was also found to be grossly dilated and the decision was made to perform a right ureterostomy. The left ureter was allowed to drain into the hydrocolpos.

THE DEFINITIVE REPAIR

- The definitive repair was performed at 10 months of age.
- A gastrostomy had been placed for feeding.
- The child was thriving.

  Preoperative imaging: Including the voiding cystourethrogram (VCUG)/cloacagram and a pelvic magnetic resonance imaging scan failed to clearly delineate the pelvic structures. At exploration this made sense in retrospect.

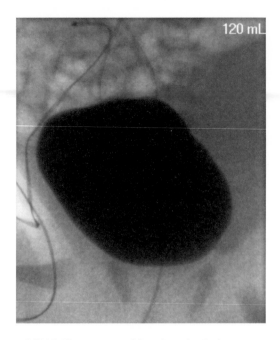

Figure 18.8 Cloacagram/VCUG. The anatomy of the urinary/vaginal system was not clearly demonstrated on the VCUG.

Primary posterior sagittal anorectoplasty: A posterior sagittal incision was made and the rectum was mobilized off the common channel to the level of the peritoneal reflection.

The presumed "common channel" was opened posteriorly, but there was no evidence of a urethra, so the exact anatomy remained unclear and a laparotomy was required.

Laparotomy: The child was then repositioned supine and a midline laparotomy was performed.

The right ureterostomy and the vaginostomy were taken down. A right nephrectomy was performed for the non-functioning dysplastic kidney. (found to have zero function of renal scan)

No bladder was identified. The ureters were found to be inserting into the hemivagina.

RECONSTRUCTION

- The vagina was reconfirmed to have a remnant of a vaginal septum.
- The right ureteral stump (from the right ureterostomy) was identified and seen to enter the right hemivagina.
- The left ureter was entering the left hemivagina, we left that in situ, making the bladder from the left hydrocolpos.
- The uterine structures were seen to enter the right hemivagina.
  - The left hemivagina was therefore reconstructed into a bladder.
  - The right hemivagina was refashioned into a tubular structure and preserved as the vagina, and pulled through.

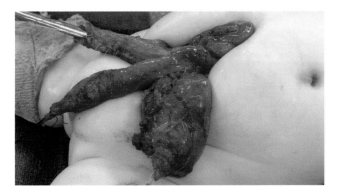

Figure 18.9 Reconstruction of the bladder and the vagina. Top structure: reconstructed vagina (with Hegar dilator in situ); middle structure: native rectum; bottom structure: neobladder created from the left hemivagina.

ANSWERS

18.1	A
18.2	A
18.3	D
18.4	C

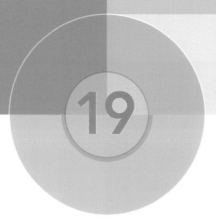

Distal colostogram: Technical points

19

When performing a high-pressure colostogram, the diagnostic components that need to be evaluated include:

A. Type of fistula
B. Relationship of fistula to the most inferior sacrococcygeal ossification
C. Absence of a fistula
D. Length of the mucous fistula
E. Distance separating fistula from expected anal position
F. All of the above

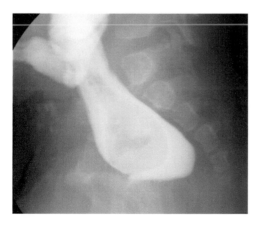

Figure 19.1 Distal colostogram. Inadequate pressure shows no fistula, but this would be the wrong conclusion.

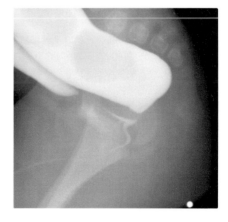

Figure 19.2 Fistulous communication is clearly demonstrated. The connection is at the "elbow" of the urethra, therefore this is a rectobulbar fistula.

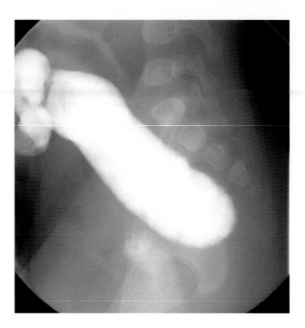

Figure 19.3 In this image of a different patient enough pressure shows a rounded distal rectum. This is consistent with a no fistula defect.

LEARNING POINTS

- The high-pressure colostogram is the most important radiologic examination to demonstrate the specific type of fistula, length of mucous fistula, the anatomic relationship of the fistula to the sacrum/coccyx, and the distance of the rectum to the expected position of the anus.
- Prior to beginning the procedure, the expected normal position of the anus is delineated with a radiopaque marker and a radiopaque ruler is placed under the patient for accurate measurements.
- A Foley catheter is inserted into the mucous fistula. Hand injection of an initial contrast bolus defines the length and relative diameter of the mucous fistula. The catheter is repositioned into a segment that is amenable to Foley balloon inflation, without the risk of perforation. The AP (anterior–posterior) view then is switched to a lateral view.
- Balloon inflation should be performed under direct fluoroscopic visualization.
- The Foley catheter is retracted proximally to lie just below the fascia until an adequate seal is obtained.
- While maintaining traction, gentle hand injection of water-soluble contrast is performed under direct fluoroscopic visualization. Injection continues until either:
  - **A:** The fistulous communication is fully delineated.
  - **B:** There is smooth and rounded configuration of the distal mucous fistula.
  - **C:** The distal colonic segment is maximally distended without demonstration of a fistula (presence of an anterior beak means incomplete distention in the presence of a fistula).

REVIEW 19.2 MULTIPLE CHOICE QUESTION

Which distal colostogram represents a bladder neck fistula?

A

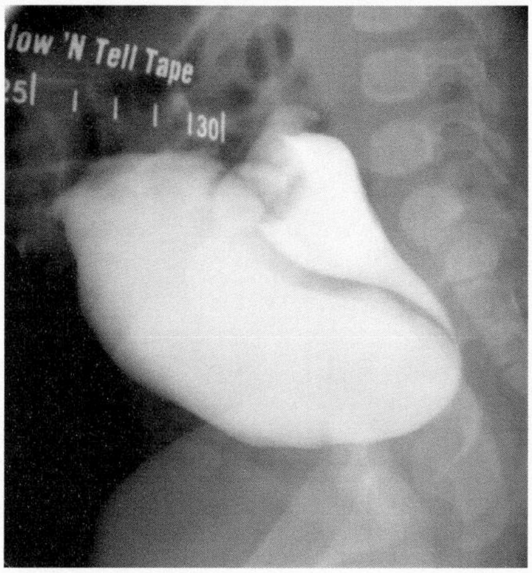

Figure 19.4

B

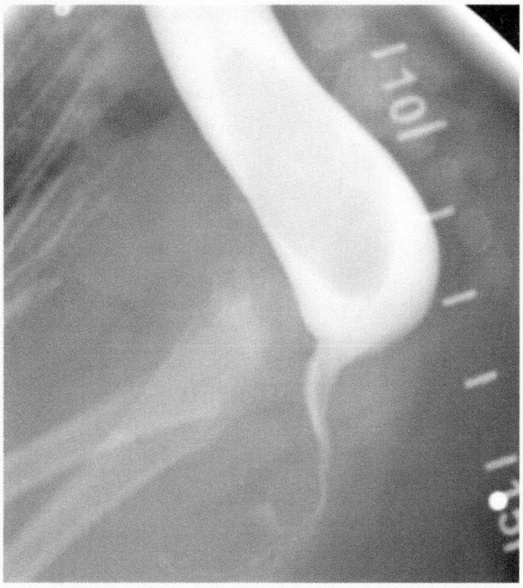

Figure 19.5

C

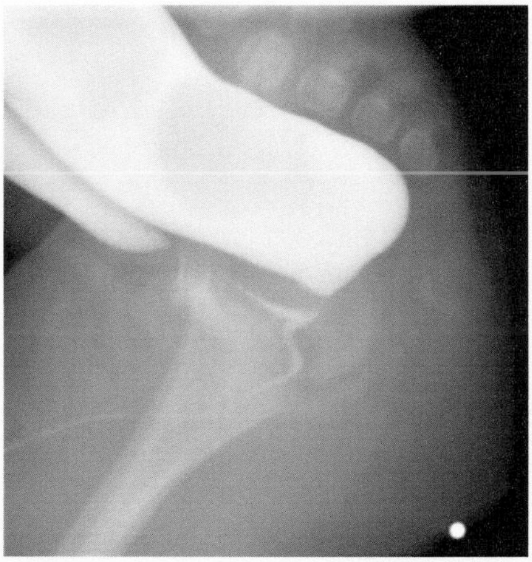

Figure 19.6

D

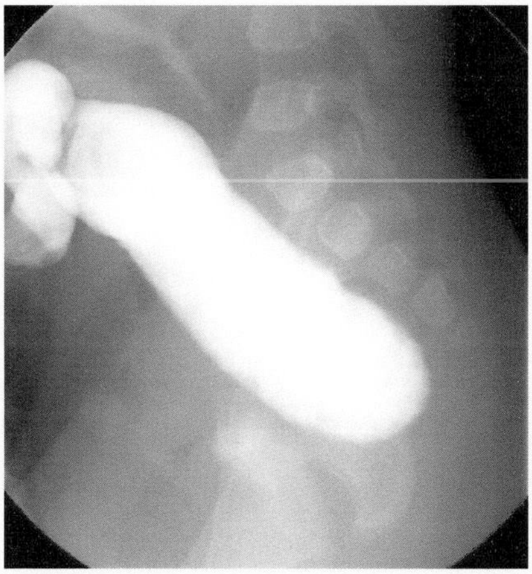

Figure 19.7

ANSWERS

19.1   F
19.2   A

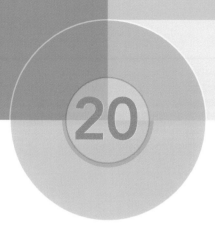

Newborn ARM: Perineal exam quiz

20

REVIEW 20.1 MULTIPLE CHOICE QUESTION

Consider the image.
What is your diagnosis?

A. Perineal fistula
B. Normal
C. Anal stenosis

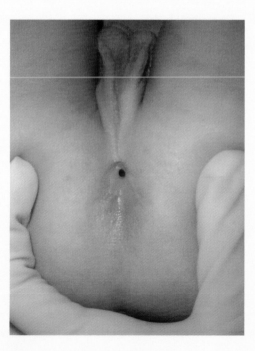

Figure 20.1 Male examination.

REVIEW 20.2 MULTIPLE CHOICE QUESTION

Consider the image.
What is your diagnosis?

A. Perineal fistula
B. Normal
C. Anal stenosis

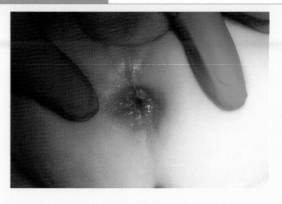

Figure 20.2 Male examination.

The position of the anus in the female infant seems to be a source of uncertainty in the pediatric surgical field, and not infrequently we are asked to give a second opinion on the matter.

The important points are:

1. Where is the anus in relation to the sphincter complex?
2. What is the size of the anus?
3. What is the length of the perineal body?

REVIEW 20.3 MULTIPLE CHOICE QUESTION

Does this female infant have an anterior anus?

A. Yes
B. No
C. Do not know

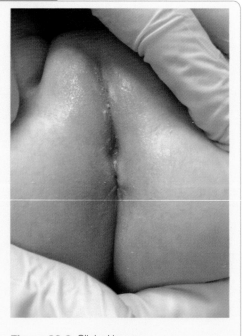

Figure 20.3 Clinical image.

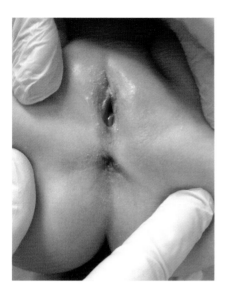

Figure 20.4 Clinical image—patient being examined. This is the same female infant. The labia and tissue lateral to the anus are flattened in order to see the anatomy better. The perineal body is adequate and the anus is positioned within the sphincter complex. By performing the maneuver, it is easier to establish the size of the perineal body. On initial examination, the perineal body appears short, but when the buttocks are separated, the perineal body is shown to be of an adequate size. The anus is then calibrated with increasing size of Hegar dilator and confirmed to be of an adequate size.

LEARNING POINTS

- It is important to spread the perineum in order to be able to establish the anatomy.

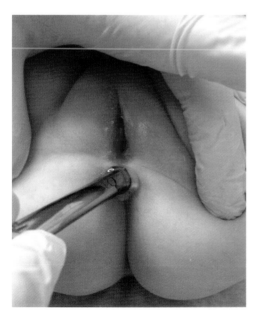

Figure 20.5 Clinical image. A size 12–13 Hegar passes without difficulty, confirming that the anus is of an adequate size.

ANSWERS

20.1	A
20.2	C
20.3	B

PART

II

ANORECTAL MALFORMATIONS— REOPERATIONS

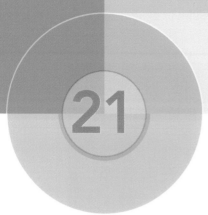
Anteriorly located anus following anoplasty: Case study

CASE HISTORY

- A 2-year-old female born with an anorectal malformation comes for assessment in the outpatient clinic. She has been adopted and there is *no previous surgical history available*.
- Her anorectal malformation was initially managed with a colostomy. She then underwent repair of the anorectal malformation and the colostomy has since been reversed.
- She is not yet potty trained.

Question 1: What further workup does this child require?

- On examination under anesthesia, she was found to have an anteriorly located anus.

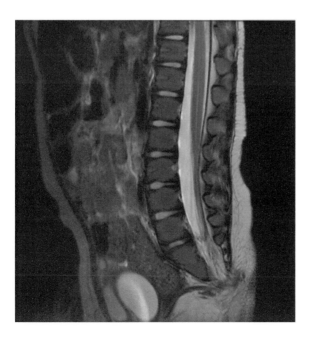

Figure 21.1 Lateral magnetic resonance (MRI) image.

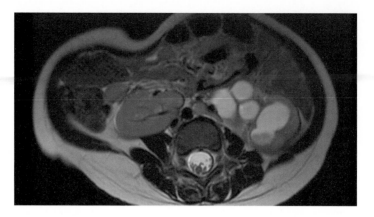

Figure 21.2 MRI. What else do you notice on the magnetic resonance imaging scan that was performed to assess the spine?

MAGNETIC RESONANCE IMAGING OF THE SPINE

- The spinal cord was found to be tethered on magnetic resonance imaging.
- The coccyx was absent.

  Does this child need spinal cord detethering?

- Neurosurgical assessment showed lower extremity weakness and the decision was made to operate for spinal cord detethering.

REPEAT NUCLEAR RENAL IMAGING

- Repeat imaging confirmed that left renal function had been preserved, with a split function of Right: 81%, Left: 19%.

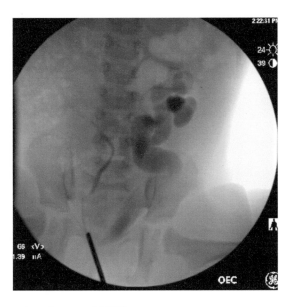

Figure 21.3 Voiding cystourethrogram (VCUG).

The VCUG demonstrates grade V reflux on the left. Cystoscopic examination revealed an ectopic left ureteral orifice at the bladder neck. What further imaging would you like to perform in order to assess the renal system?

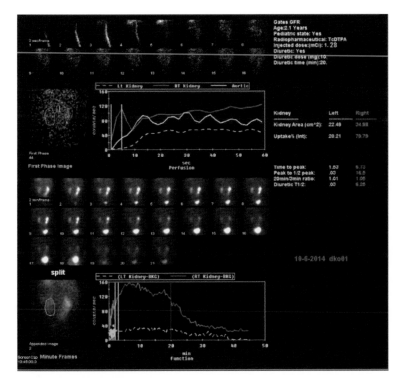

Figure 21.4 Nuclear renal scan—Right 80%, Left 20%.

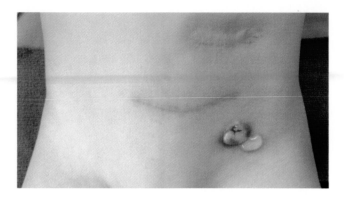

Figure 21.5 Cutaneous ureterostomy was performed.

LEARNING POINTS

- When the original surgery and the type of anorectal malformation is unknown, the child requires a thorough workup, including EUA and assessment of the spine, sacrum, and renal system.
    - In this child a number of important factors were found:
        - Misplaced anus
        - Tethered spinal cord requiring release
        - Grade V reflux with poor-functioning left kidney
        - Ectopic ureter
- Ultimately a redo PSARP was performed to locate the anus within the sphincter mechanism. The cord was detethered. And, the left ureter was reimplanted.

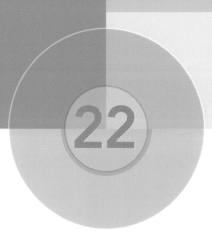

Anorectal malformation—Postoperative problem: Case study

22

CASE HISTORY

- 3-year-old male
- Anorectal malformation with previously repaired bladder neck fistula
- Not potty trained for urine

EXAMINATION UNDER ANESTHESIA OF THE ANUS

- Posteriorly mislocated anus, no anal stricture

MAGNETIC RESONANCE IMAGING OF THE SPINE

- Normal
- No evidence of a pre-sacral mass

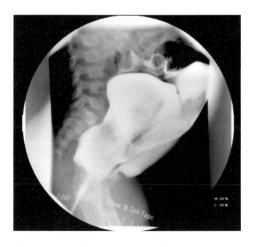

Figure 22.1 Contrast enema. What does the contrast enema show?

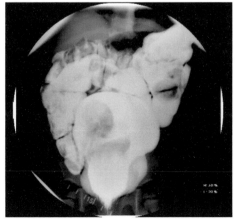

Figure 22.2 Dilated rectum and colon, compressing the bladder anteriorly.

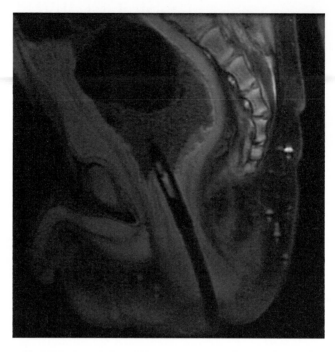

Figure 22.3 Magnetic resonance imaging of the spine. No evidence of a pre-sacral mass or a remnant of the original fistula.

LEARNING POINTS

- The anatomy in this child is not optimal (mislocated anus with rectum outside of the sphincter mechanism) and he will not successfully potty train. The dilated distal colon occurred likely due to years of inadequate management of constipation. He will require a redo procedure in the future to maximize his potential for future bowel control, but it is potentially possible to keep him clean with an enema regimen as a "first step."
- When he is older and after the anatomy has been corrected, he may be able to have spontaneous bowel movements with/without laxatives, in particular considering the evidence of a good sacrum on the contrast enema **(Figure 22.1)**.

The patient therefore underwent the bowel management enema program (see below).

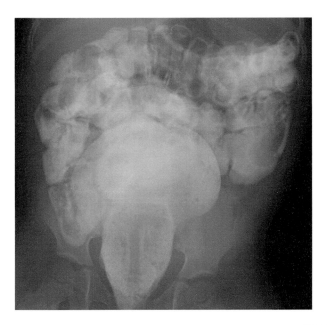

Figure 22.4 Bowel management radiograph. Day 1: Bowel management program (BMP). Needs enemas to clear the rectum of stool before considering laxatives. Initial regimen selected based on this image was saline 500 mL and glycerin 20 mL.

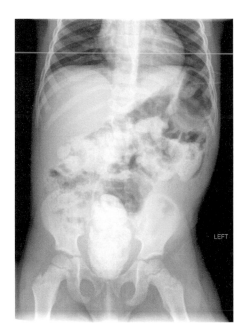

Figure 22.5 Day 3: Despite rectal enemas, the rectum is still loaded with stool and contrast material is evident. He was complaining of pain with the initial regimen and this was therefore changed to saline 500 mL and Castile soap 27 mL.

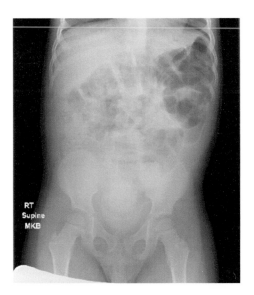

Figure 22.6 The colon is more clean, but not completely empty despite a strong enema. He will continue with this regimen for now. Consideration is made of removal of some of the dilated sigmoid with the Malone procedure to make the antegrade flush easier.

LEARNING POINTS

- The patient succeeded with the bowel management program with rectal enemas. He will undergo redo primary posterior sagittal anorectoplasty with Malone appendicostomy to correct the anatomy and provide a route for antegrade enemas.
- When more mature, he would be a suitable candidate for a laxative trial to see if his now corrected anatomy will enable him to achieve continence without the need for mechanical emptying provided by a daily flush.

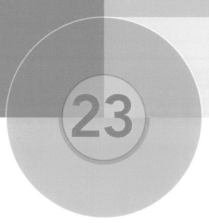
Anorectal malformation—Rectal prolapse and soiling: Case study

CASE HISTORY

- This is a case of a 3-year-old girl who is known to have undergone a primary posterior sagittal anorectoplasty (PSARP) as an infant for an anorectal malformation.
- She has no scars on the abdomen to suggest that she has had a previous colostomy and you therefore suspect that her original malformation was a perineal fistula or a vestibular fistula.
- She has come to see you because she has a rectal prolapse and is having difficulties with potty training.

What else would you like to know about this child?

You decide that you need to perform a number of investigations.
Explain to the parents the investigations that you think are necessary and the rationale.

REVIEW 23.1 MULTIPLE CHOICE QUESTION

What is the most accurate description of the sacrum in this radiograph?

A. Normal sacrum
B. S1–S2 present
C. Sacral agenesis
D. Hemisacrum

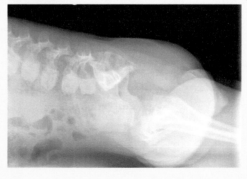

Figure 23.1 Lateral x-ray of sacrum.

REVIEW 23.2 MULTIPLE CHOICE QUESTION

What is most concerning from this contrast enema?

A. Proximal bowel dilatation indicating a stricture
B. Severe constipation accounting for the rectal prolapse
C. Nothing of concern on this study
D. Widening of the space between the spine and rectum

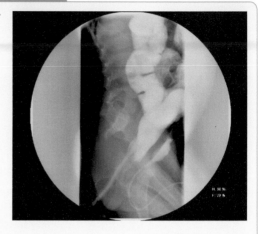

Figure 23.2

MAGNETIC RESONANCE IMAGING RESULT

The magnetic resonance imaging scan confirms your suspicion that there is a pre-sacral mass (measuring $3.5 \times 2.5 \times 2.2$ cm) as suggested on the contrast enema. There is also tethering of the spinal cord at L4/L5.

RENAL ULTRASOUND RESULT

Left hydronephrosis.

What further urological investigations are required?

REVIEW 23.3 MULTIPLE CHOICE QUESTION

What does the VCUG demonstrate?

A. Right vesicoureteral reflux (VUR)
B. Normal
C. Bilateral VUR
D. Left VUR

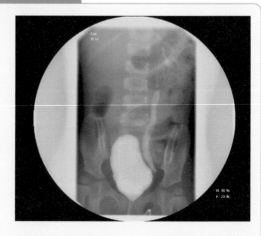

Figure 23.3

EXAMINATION UNDER ANESTHESIA (EUA)/ CYSTOVAGINOSCOPY

Trabeculated, low-capacity bladder. Narrow introitus and short vaginal vault. Mislocated anus.

URODYNAMICS

High-pressure/low-volume bladder.

Based on the information provided, the further management this child require includes:

1. Redo primary posterior sagittal anorectoplasty, vaginal replacement
2. Resection of pre-sacral mass
3. Detethering of the spinal cord
4. Intermittent catheterization to protect upper renal tracts and consideration for Mitrofanoff procedure
5. Appendicostomy for bowel management given poor sacrum and tethered cord, and reduced capacity for voluntary bowel movements

ANSWERS

23.1	B
23.2	D
23.3	D

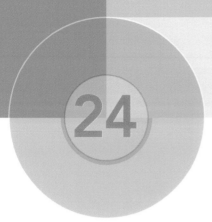

Anorectal malformation—
Long-term: Case study

24

CASE HISTORY

- This is a long-term case study of a child born with an anorectal malformation and VACTERL association:
  - Tracheo-esophageal fistula (TEF)/esophageal atresia (EA).
  - Hydronephrosis.
  - Lipoma of the spinal cord.
  - Atrial septal defect.
- He was managed in the newborn period with repair of the TEF/EA and the anorectal malformation was managed with a colostomy and mucous fistula.

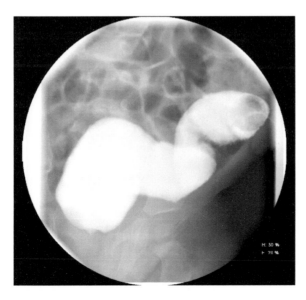

Figure 24.1 Distal colostogram. A–P view.

REVIEW 24.1 MULTIPLE CHOICE QUESTION

What type of anorectal malformation does the patient have based on the images shown?

A. No fistula
B. Rectobulbar fistula
C. Rectoprostatic fistula
D. Bladder neck fistula
E. Inadequate study

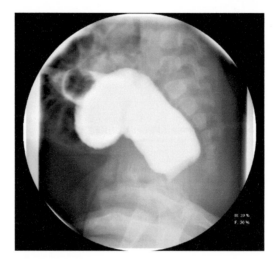

Figure 24.2 Lateral view of distal colostogram.

LATERAL

- The reason for performing the distal loop colostogram is to demonstrate the position of the distal rectum and fistula (if present). This is only achieved if a high-pressure study is performed. **Figure 24.2 shows a flat distal rectum at the level of the pubococcygeal line, which is indicative of a low-pressure (inadequate) study.**
- On occasion, no fistula is present, a malformation that is most commonly seen in children with trisomy 21, but the distal rectum should be bulging under pressure before the surgeon can make this diagnosis.
- If the position of the fistula and the location of the distal rectum is known, the surgeon can more safely find the distal rectum intra-operatively.
- The surgeon can also decide whether the definitive surgical repair is possible through a posterior sagittal approach alone or whether it will require a laparotomy/laparoscopic-assisted procedure.
- Based on the colostogram demonstrated, the operative surgeon has not gained enough useful information. The colostogram has not demonstrated the position of the fistula. If the primary posterior sagittal anorectoplasty (PSARP) is performed, it will be done "blindly," risking damage to the urinary tract.
- However, the patient underwent a posterior sagittal anorectoplasty at 1 year of age without further imaging.

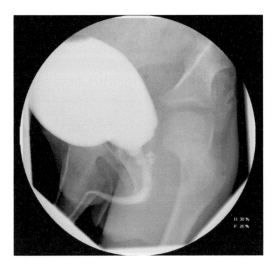

Figure 24.3 VCUG. What is your interpretation of the VCUG?

- The child was reviewed at the age of 4–5 years with problems of fecal and urinary incontinence.
- The child underwent a VCUG as part of routine workup.
- **Why was the VCUG performed?**

On the posterior wall of the urethra is an out-pouching of contrast, likely to represent a retained segment of distal rectum that was not fully excised at the time of initial repair. This would be a remnant of the original fistula (ROOF).

This is at risk of malignant change and needs to be excised as it can cause urinary and mucous dribbling and be a nidus for stone formation. Also if he is difficult to catheterize because of this outpouching that will limit his urologic care.

- Of note in the past medical history, a *lipoma of the filum terminale* was seen on spinal magnetic resonance imaging (MRI) at 1 year of age. The child has presented with fecal and urinary incontinence, and on neurosurgical review was noted to have lower back pain and pain in the back of the legs during growth spurts.
- A second MRI of the spine was therefore performed at the age of 4 years, which again demonstrated the fatty filum terminale.
- Clinically, the patient was showing features consistent with a tethered cord and is awaiting tethered cord release.
- Constipation has been a concern and he underwent evaluation for this to rule out the anatomical problems with the anoplasty (e.g., a stricture). Rectal enemas have been attempted, but patient compliance was an issue and therefore a cecostomy for antegrade enemas was placed.

EXAMINATION UNDER ANESTHESIA OF THE ANUS

- Rectal prolapse.
- *No evidence of stricture* despite the appearance on the contrast enema of a grossly dilated rectosigmoid.

CYSTOSCOPY

- Remnant of the original fistula (ROOF).
- *Urethra was not catheterizable.*

Why is the rectosigmoid so dilated?

1. Inherent dysmotility associated with anorectal malformations
2. Inadequate constipation management during the first few years of life

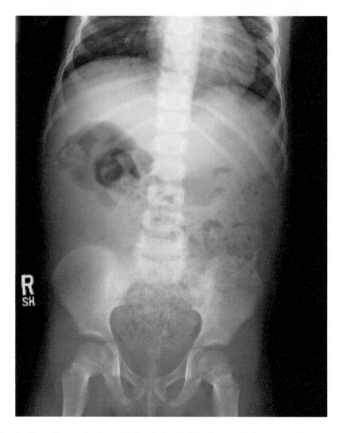

Figure 24.4 Evaluation of constipation. Plain abdominal radiograph demonstrating gross constipation. Please see next image.

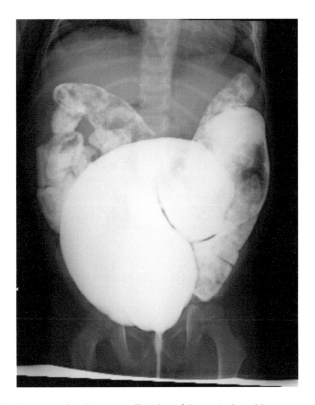

Figure 24.5 Contrast enema showing gross dilatation of the rectosigmoid.

MANAGEMENT

1. Tethered cord release (symptomatic).
2. Redo PSARP.
   - Rectal prolapse repair and resection of ROOF due to potential for urinary tract infection, stone formation, malignant transformation, and to allow for a smooth urethra and intermittent catheterization if needed.
3. Bowel management.
   - Enemas (offer option for retrograde enemas via cecostomy).
   Note: Cecostomy done as initial step, to preserve the appendix for use later as Mitrofanoff, or as a split appendix for Malone/Mitrofanoff.
4. Urological management.
   - Does this child require clean intermittent catheterization to empty bladder? Is the urethra easily catheterizable?
   - Renal tract USS.
5. Reassess bowel function and full urological assessment.
   - He may require a combination of:
     - Colonic resection.
     - Malone/neo-Malone.
     - Bladder augmentation ± Mitrofanoff. (which could potentially use the dilated sigmoid)

LEARNING POINTS

1. The presenting bowel and urinary symptoms can be secondary to a neurological concern (i.e., tethered cord) and this must not be overlooked.
2. The child requires a tethered cord release. The bowel and urological system need to be managed in the interim and reassessed after the release.
3. Rectal enemas were attempted in this child. However, they were not tolerated due to his age and therefore a cecostomy may be a good alternative.
4. The child needs a redo PSARP to repair the rectal prolapse and the ROOF can be excised at the same time. This may also help with catheterization of the urethra.
5. Postoperatively, the bowel and urological system can be reassessed.
   - The child may fail to empty the grossly dilated colon with enemas and may require a colonic resection.
   - If he is found to require a bladder augmentation, this can be done in the same sitting, with the resected colon being used for the augment.
   - The cecostomy can be refashioned as a Malone.
   - A Mitrofanoff can be formed with the appendix being split.

ANSWER

24.1   E

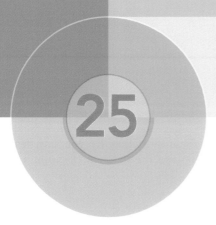

25

Postoperative complication—Mislocated anus: Case study

CASE HISTORY

- A 3-year-old girl comes to see you in the outpatient clinic.
- She has had a previous operation to repair an anorectal malformation with a rectovestibular fistula.
- The parents have not been able to potty train her.
- You decide to perform an examination under anesthesia of the anus with electrical stimulation
- Figure 25.1 shows your examination findings.

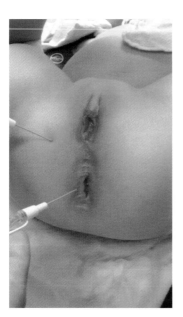

Figure 25.1 View of the anus.

REVIEW 25.1 MULTIPLE CHOICE QUESTION

What is your assessment?

A. Anus positioned too close to the vagina (anterior mislocation)

B. Normal findings

C. Anus positioned too far towards the coccyx (posterior mislocation)

- This patient also has a history of
  - Hemisacrum
  - Tethered cord release
  - Sacral ratio is 0.43

What is your prediction of fecal continence based on the information that you have been provided with (i.e., the type of anorectal malformation and the status of the spine and sacrum)?

REVIEW 25.2 MULTIPLE CHOICE QUESTION

How are you going to manage this patient?

A. Rectal enemas

B. Appendicostomy

C. Redo primary posterior sagittal anorectoplasty to relocate the anus

D. Redo primary posterior sagittal anorectoplasty to relocate the anus and appendicostomy

E. Laxatives

LEARNING POINTS

- The anus is posteriorly mislocated outside the muscle complex, which will contribute to her inability to potty train, and she requires redo surgery.
- Her continence potential is reduced by the fact that she has a history of tethered cord and her sacral ratio is 0.43.
- She is likely to require enemas to achieve social fecal continence (rectal or antegrade).
- In future, she may be able to transition to laxatives, as once her anus is properly located within the sphincter mechanism, only then can she realize her continence potential.

ANSWERS

25.1	C
25.2	D

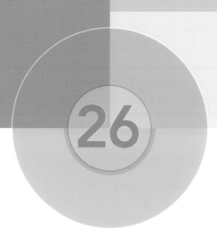

Postoperative complication—Female anorectal malformation: Case study

26

The patients shown in the photos below have both undergone previous surgery to repair an anorectal malformation.

Please consider the postoperative images below. What do you notice on clinical examination?

ON EXAMINATION

Figure 26.1

- The urethra and the vagina appear normal.
- The perineal body is not adequate and the anus is too narrow.
- The anus is stenotic and not well centered within the sphincter complex.

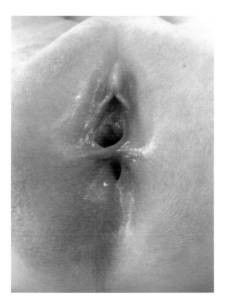

Figure 26.1 View of perineum.

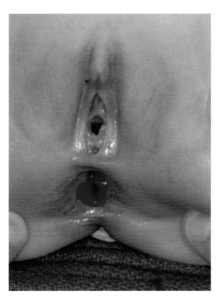

Figure 26.2 View of perineum.

- There is no posterior sagittal incision from previous surgery, suggesting that this incision was not used. There may, therefore have been previous inadequate mobilization of the anterior rectum from the posterior wall of the vagina at the original operation.

Figure 26.2

- The urethra and the vagina appear normal.
- There is a remnant of the rectovestibular fistula (i.e., the original distal rectum was left behind when a more proximal segment of rectum was mobilized for the anoplasty.
- The anus does not appear to be well centered within the sphincter complex.

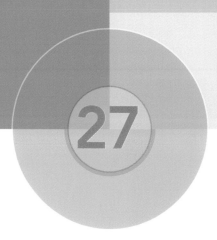

Postoperative complication— No medical history in an ARM patient: Case study

27

You see a 3-year-old male child with a past medical history of an anorectal malformation. He has a scar on the abdomen from a previous colostomy that has been reversed. On examination of the perineum, he has evidence of a previous rectal repair. He is adopted and there is no past medical or surgical history available to you when you take over the medical care.

Question 1: What work-up does this child need?

Answer 1

Genitourinary evaluation:

- Renal US ± assessment for vesicoureteral reflux
- Urodynamics if there is evidence to suggest poor bladder compliance and emptying.

Spinal evaluation:

- Vertebral radiographs to assess for hemivertebrae and scoliosis.
- Spinal magnetic resonance imaging to assess for occult spinal dysraphism/tethered cord.

Sacral evaluation:

- Sacral radiographs to assess for hemisacrum suggestive of pre-sacral mass (± pelvic magnetic resonance imaging).

REVIEW 27.1 MULTIPLE CHOICE QUESTION

Given all of the information that you have been provided with, what is the likely original malformation?

A. Perineal fistula
B. Rectobulbar fistula
C. Rectoprostatic fistula
D. Bladder neck fistula
E. B, C, or D could be correct given the prior colostomy scar.

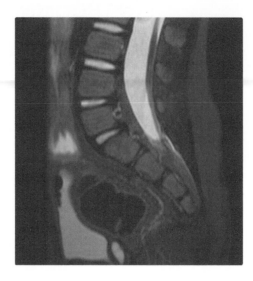

Figure 27.1 Magnetic resonance imaging scan of the spine.

- Sacral radiograph to calculate the sacral ratio, which can assist in predicting the continence potential.

Question 2: What abnormality do you see on the magnetic resonance imaging scan?

Answer 2: The magnetic resonance imaging scan shows a possible ROOF or a congenital prostatic utricle. The child will need further cystoscopic evaluation to assess the anatomy. There is no evidence of a pre-sacral mass. The trajectory of the pull-through appears centered within the sphincters.

LEARNING POINTS

- If you have no past medical history, the child needs a full VACTERL screen to identify spinal, sacral, and renal pathology [1].
- If a male child has evidence of a previous colostomy, then it is likely that the child had a rectourethral fistula (rectobulbar or rectoprostatic) or a bladder neck fistula. From the magnetic resonance imaging scan of the pelvis, it appears that the remnant of the original fistula (ROOF) is at the rectoprostatic level in this case.

REFERENCE

1. Lane VA, Skerritt C, Wood RJ, Reck C, Hewitt GD, McCracken KA, Jayanthi VR et al. A standardized approach for the assessment and treatment of internationally adopted children with a previously repaired anorectal malformation (ARM). *J Pediatr Surg* 2016, 51(11):1864–1870.

ANSWER

27.1   E

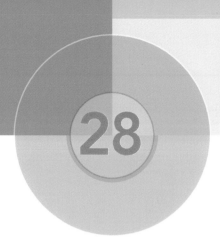

Postoperative complication—Recto-perineal fistula: Case study

28

CASE HISTORY

- A surgeon has performed a posterior sagittal anorectoplasty on a male infant with a recto-perineal fistula.
- They did not pass a urethral catheter at the start of the procedure.
- The following day, the nurses report that there is urine draining from around the anoplasty.
- Consider the questions below.

1. **What are your concerns considering the history given from the nursing staff?**

   Answer 1: The most likely explanation is that there has been a urethral injury intra-operatively, explaining the leakage of urine from the anoplasty site. This is likely to have occurred due to failure to catheterize the patient before the operation and an anterior rectal wall dissection that inadvertently injured the urethra. Preoperatively, a urethral catheter should be inserted in all cases to assist in the identification and preservation of the urethra, and a meticulous anterior rectal wall dissection should be carried out.

2. **How are you going to manage this patient?**

   Answer 2: There are several options available to you to manage the urethral injury; however, the best option is probably to attempt to pass a cystoscope[*] and a urethral catheter and also consider placing a suprapubic catheter. Leave the urethral catheter and the suprapubic catheter for 4–6 weeks, with the aim being to allow the urethral injury to heal.

   Following this, remove the urethral catheter and perform a void trial by clamping the suprapubic catheter.

3. **What are the long-term implications?**

   Answer 3: Urethral stricture or acquired atresia, both of which may require a redo procedure.

---

[*] If at cystoscopy the urethra cannot be passed successfully to the bladder, a suprapubic bladder catheter should be inserted and the child will likely require a redo primary posterior sagittal anorectoplasty with urethral dilations or urethral repair.

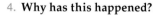
4. **Why has this happened?**

Answer 4: This happens most commonly when the urethra has not been catheterized preoperatively and the anterior rectal wall dissection is too deep and invades into the posterior urethra. In rectourethral fistula cases, urethral injuries can occur, when the surgeon has failed to perform an adequate distal colostogram preoperatively to identify the position of the rectum, a urinary tract injury is more likely to occur.

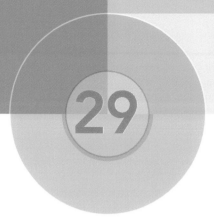

Postoperative complication— Redo surgery: Case study

29

CASE HISTORY

An 8-year-old boy has had a previous posterior sagittal anorectoplasty for repair of a recto-prostatic fistula and has been referred to you for ongoing care. He has problems with fecal incontinence and the family would like a second opinion. You perform an examination under anesthesia and the findings are shown in Figure 29.1.

What is your opinion? Answer the multiple choice questions below.

REVIEW 29.1 MULTIPLE CHOICE QUESTION

The anus (in relation to the muscle complex) is:

A. Posteriorly mislocated in the midline
B. Posteriorly and laterally mislocated to the left
C. Posteriorly and laterally mislocated to the right
D. Normal
E. Anteriorly mislocated in the midline
F. Anteriorly mislocated to the left

REVIEW 29.2 MULTIPLE CHOICE QUESTION

How would you manage this child?

A. Cecostomy/Malone appendicostomy for antegrade flushes
B. Redo anoplasty
C. Increase the dose of laxatives
D. End colostomy
E. Redo anoplasty and consider cecostomy/Malone appendicostomy

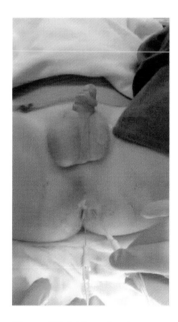

Figure 29.1 View of perineum.

LEARNING POINTS

- This child's anus is posteriorly mislocated and is lying outside of the sphincter complex.
- He will be unable to squeeze the anus closed as it is lying outside the muscle complex, which is one of the major contributing factors to his fecal incontinence.
- The other points to consider are:
  - His spine needs to be assessed for associated tethered cord, which could also affect his continence potential.
  - His original malformation was a rectoprostatic fistula and therefore his potential for continence is less than that of a "lower" malformation, such as a bulbar or perineal fistula.
  - At this age, he would benefit from a reliable method of bowel management (e.g., cecostomy/Malone appendicostomy).

When confident and mature enough after a successful redo and therefore improved anatomy he can undergo a laxative trial and, if he succeeds, the antegrade flushes can be discontinued.

ANSWERS

29.1   A
29.2   E

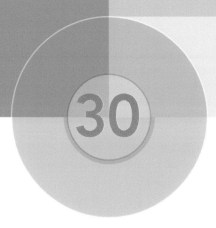

Postoperative complication: Case study

30

CASE HISTORY

- A 3-year-old boy who had a previous posterior sagittal anorectoplasty for a rectobulbar fistula and has been referred to you for ongoing care.
- He is having problems with potty training. In order to evaluate the child, you perform an examination under anesthesia. The sacral ratio is 0.72 and the spine is normal.

The findings of the EUA are shown in Figure 30.1.

REVIEW 30.1 MULTIPLE CHOICE QUESTION

The anus (in relation to the muscle complex) is:

A. Posteriorly mislocated in the midline
B. Posteriorly and laterally mislocated to the left
C. Posteriorly and laterally mislocated to the right
D. Normal
E. Anteriorly mislocated in the midline
F. Anteriorly mislocated to the left

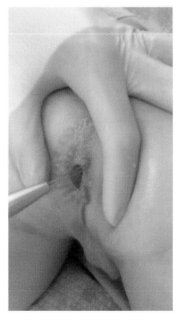

Figure 30.1 View of the perineum, in prone position.

REVIEW 30.2 MULTIPLE CHOICE QUESTION

This patient has failed attempts at potty training and is incontinent of stool.

How are you going to manage this patient?

A. Do nothing at this stage and re-examine when 5–6 years old.

B. Redo primary posterior sagittal anorectoplasty to reposition the anus and subsequent bowel management as required.

C. Bowel management with enemas to keep socially clean.

D. Cecostomy for bowel washouts to keep socially clean.

ANSWERS

30.1   A
30.2   B

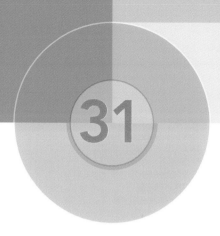

Redo surgery in anorectal malformations

There have been significant advances in the care of children with anorectal malformations in recent years; however, there continues to be significant morbidity associated with repair of the various conditions.

Many of these problems are a consequence of the underlying congenital malformation that requires careful management; however, a significant proportion is iatrogenic and potentially avoidable.

Efforts continue to improve the education of pediatric surgeons around the world, and there have been many publications in the literature with the goal being to share experience, ideas, and lessons learned. The aim of this section is to demonstrate some of the common postoperative complications seen.

We often wonder why this field is so fraught with technically related morbidity. We surmise that surgeons have limited experience with the entire spectrum of defects and, if there is a technical misadventure, the impact of that posterior urethral injury or anal mislocation, for example, may not manifest as a problem until several years later. At that point, the surgeon may not have any recollection of the technical issues surrounding the case and therefore may have no appreciation of the need to alter their technique for future cases. All surgeons will encounter complications secondary to infection and patient disease. The following complications, however, have occurred because of one of the following:

a. Failure to perform/or correctly execute radiological investigations to establish the anatomy and aid in surgical planning
b. Failure to recognize the underlying precise anatomy of the congenital malformation leading to subsequent poor surgical decision making
c. Inadequate mobilization of structures and failure to preserve blood supply leading to tension and poor healing, strictures, fistulae, and acquired atresia of structures

It is key to identify where the primary surgeons faltered in terms of the following:

1. Diagnosis
2. Decision making
3. Investigations
4. Operative techniques

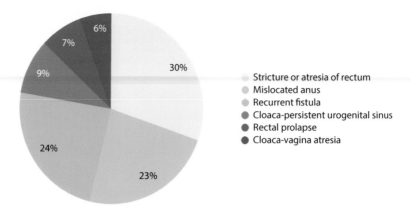

Figure 31.1 Anorectal malformations: Indication for redo surgery (Pena A et al. *J Ped Surg* 2007; 42: 318–325).

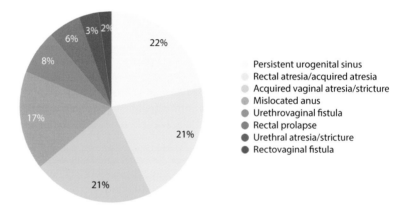

Figure 31.2 Cloacal malformations: Indication for redo surgery (Levitt MA et al. *J Ped Surg* 2011; 46: 1250–1255).

The common complications following anorectal malformation repair include:

1. Stricture or acquired atresia of the rectum
2. Mislocated rectum outside the sphincter mechanism
3. Fistulae—recurrent, persistent, or acquired
4. Remnant of original fistula
5. Persistent urogenital sinus in cloacal malformations
6. Rectal prolapse
7. Vaginal atresia
8. Urethral atresia or stricture
9. Persistent cloaca

REFERENCES

Levitt MA et al. Pitfalls and challenges of cloacal repair: How to reduce the need for reoperations. *J Ped Surg* 2011; 46: 1250–1255.

Pena A et al. Reoperations in anorectal malformations. *J Ped Surg* 2007; 42: 318–325.

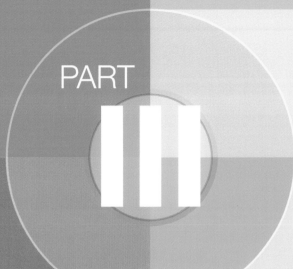

PART III

HIRSCHSPRUNG DISEASE (HD)—PRIMARY

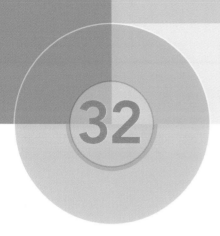

Hirschsprung disease newborn algorithm

MANAGEMENT ALGORITHMS

NEWBORN INFANT

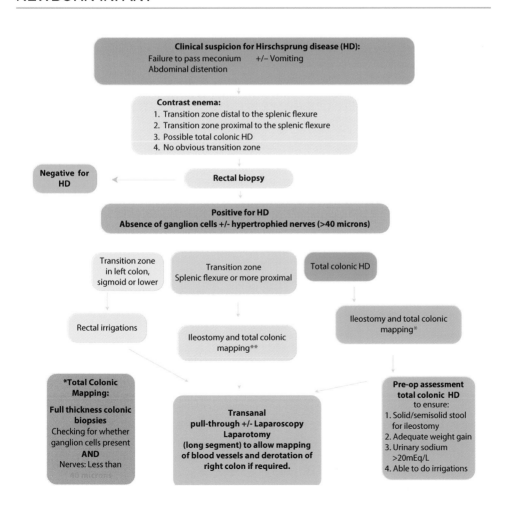

Clinical suspicion for Hirschsprung disease (HD):
Failure to pass meconium   +/– Vomiting
Abdominal distention

Contrast enema:
1. Transition zone distal to the splenic flexure
2. Transition zone proximal to the splenic flexure
3. Possible total colonic HD
4. No obvious transition zone

Rectal biopsy

Negative for HD

Positive for HD
Absence of ganglion cells +/- hypertrophied nerves (>40 microns)

Transition zone in left colon, sigmoid or lower

Transition zone Splenic flexure or more proximal

Total colonic HD

Rectal irrigations

Ileostomy and total colonic mapping**

Ileostomy and total colonic mapping*

***Total Colonic Mapping:**

Full thickness colonic biopsies
Checking for whether ganglion cells present
AND
Nerves: Less than 40 microns

Transanal pull-through +/- Laparoscopy Laparotomy (long segment) to allow mapping of blood vessels and derotation of right colon if required.

Pre-op assessment total colonic HD
to ensure:
1. Solid/semisolid stool for ileostomy
2. Adequate weight gain
3. Urinary sodium >20mEq/L
4. Able to do irrigations

LEARNING POINTS

- Hypertrophied nerves are considered to be over 40 μm.
- Leveling colostomy is dependent on high-quality frozen section analysis and is not as reliable when taking biopsies proximal to the splenic flexure. We therefore recommend, in such a case, total colonic mapping (biopsies can then be assessed on permanent section) with formation of an ileostomy.

Enterocolitis scoring system

CASE HISTORY 1

- You are seeing a child with a previous history of Hirschsprung-associated enterocolitis (HAEC). Currently, the child has a history of diarrhea with foul smelling stool, has a distended abdomen, and the abdominal radiograph shows multiple air fluid levels. Laboratory results demonstrate leukocytosis.

CASE HISTORY 2

- You review another child who has no previous history of HAEC. On review, the child has been suffering from foul smelling and bloody stool. On physical examination, the abdomen is distended, there is an explosive release of stool on digital rectal examination, and the child has a fever. The radiology demonstrates pneumatosis and dilated loops.

REVIEW 33.1 MULTIPLE CHOICE QUESTION

What is the HAEC score for case history 1?

A. 7
B. 3
C. 15
D. 5

REVIEW 33.2 MULTIPLE CHOICE QUESTION

What is the HAEC score for case history 2?

A. 5
B. 10
C. 3
D. 8

See below and the HAEC scoring system for further information.

Table 33.1 HAEC score (the Langer score)

Criteria	Score
History	
Diarrhea with explosive stool	2
Diarrhea with foul smelling stool	2
Diarrhea with bloody stool	1
Previous history of HAEC	1
Physical examination	
Explosive discharge of gas and stool on rectal examination	2
Distended abdomen	2
Decreased peripheral perfusion	1
Lethargy	1
Fever	1
Radiology	
Multiple air fluid levels	1
Dilated loops of bowel	1
Sawtooth appearance with irregular mucosal lining	1
Cut-off sign in the rectosigmoid with absence of distal air	1
Pneumatosis	1
Laboratory	
Leukocytosis	1
Shift to the left	1
Total	20
HAEC	≥10

Source: Adapted from Pastor AC et al. *J Ped Surg* 2009; 44: 251–256.

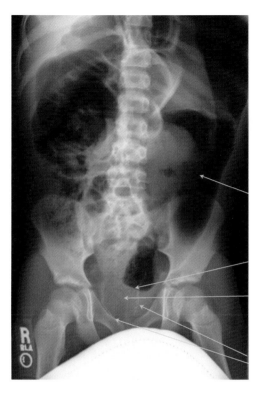

This patient has had a previous Duhamel pull-through

The radiological features of HAEC are shown:

• Dilated loops of bowel

• Cut-off sign in rectosigmoid

• Absence of distal gas distally

• Staple lines from Duhamel pull-through.

Figure 33.1 Abdominal x-ray.

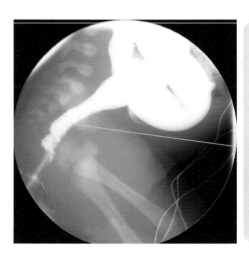

This is the contrast enema of a newborn infant demonstrating the transition zone

Sawtooth appearance of rectum on contrast enema consistent with HAEC

Figure 33.2 Contrast enema.

REFERENCE

Pastor AC et al. Development of a standardized definition of Hirschsprung's associated enterocolitis: A Delphi Analysis. *J Ped Surg* 2009; 44: 251–256.

ANSWERS

33.1   A
33.2   B

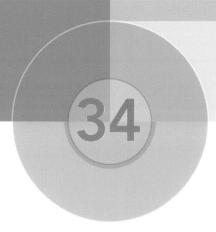

Genetics: Case study

34

- The family of a 3-year-old girl with Hirschsprung disease comes to see you in the clinic.
- They mention to you that they are planning for a second child and want to know the risks of this infant also having Hirschsprung disease.

REVIEW 34.1 MULTIPLE CHOICE QUESTION

What is Carter's paradox?

A. The highest recurrence risk is in the sister of a girl with short segment Hirschsprung disease.

B. The highest recurrence risk is in the brother of a girl with long segment Hirschsprung disease.

C. The highest recurrence risk is in the sister of a boy with long segment Hirschsprung disease.

D. The highest recurrence risk is in the brother of a boy with short segment Hirschsprung disease.

LEARNING POINTS

- The incidence of Hirschsprung disease is 1:5000; however, the overall recurrence risk in siblings is 4%, given a relative risk of 200 compared to the general population.
- In isolated Hirschsprung disease, the *length* of the aganglionosis and *sex* of the children affects the risk of recurrence. The highest risk is for the brother of a girl with long segment Hirschsprung disease.
- Table 34.1 summarizes the risks.

Table 34.1 Epidemiology and recurrence risk of Hirschsprung disease

Sex and length of aganglionosis in proband	Risk of recurrence in a brother (%)	Risk of recurrence in a sister (%)
Male + short segment	5	1
Male + long segment	17	13
Female + short segment	5	3
Female + long segment	33	9

REVIEW 34.2 MULTIPLE CHOICE QUESTION

Which chromosomal abnormality is most commonly associated with Hirschsprung disease?

A. Mosaic trisomy 8
B. 13q22.1–32.1 interstitial deletion
C. Trisomy 21
D. 10q11.2 interstitial deletion
E. Trisomy 13

LEARNING POINTS

- Chromosomal abnormalities are reported in 12% of Hirschsprung disease patients. Trisomy 21 is responsible for over 90% of chromosomal anomalies and affects up to 10% of Hirschsprung disease patients. However, it is not clear whether overexpression of gene(s) on chromosome 21 is responsible for the development of Hirschsprung disease or whether other predisposing genes are involved. The predominance of short segment Hirschsprung disease is greater in this group than in the general population.
- 10q11.2 interstitial deletion was observed in a few patients with either long segment or total colonic aganglionosis and helped to identify the first known predisposing gene, *RET*, which codes for a tyrosine kinase receptor expressed in neural crest-derived cells. There have been over 100 different mutations identified in Hirschsprung disease patients. *RET* is a proto-oncogene and certain activating mutations account for disease in multiple endocrine neoplasia (MEN) 2A syndrome, which can co-occur in some families with Hirschsprung disease. However, a *RET* mutation is only identified in 50% of familial and 15%–20% of sporadic cases of Hirschsprung disease.
- 13q22.1–32.1 interstitial deletion was found *de novo* in several patients with Hirschsprung disease. It contains a gene coding for endothelin receptor B (ENDRB). The piebald-lethal murine model of Hirschsprung disease consists of ENDRB-knockout mice. ENDRB mutations have been found in approximately 5% of Hirschsprung disease patients.
- There have been case reports of mosaic trisomy 8 associated with Hirschsprung disease.
- There is no known associations with trisomy 13.

Which syndromes are frequently associated with Hirschsprung disease?

A. MEN 2A, Shah–Waardenburg, central hypoventilation syndrome

B. MEN 2A, Bardet–Biedl, Williams

C. Shah–Waardenburg, CHARGE (coloboma, heart defects, atresia choanae, retarded growth, genital abnormality, and ear abnormality), Silver–Russell

D. Dandy–Walker, Di George, Kabuki

LEARNING POINTS

- Up to 18% of Hirschsprung disease patients have an associated syndrome, some of which have an autosomal dominant pattern of inheritance. This highlights the importance of careful assessment by a clinical geneticist if there is any suggestion of dysmorphology.
- MEN 2A, Shah–Waardenburg, and central hypoventilation syndromes are all neurocristopathies that are frequently associated with Hirschsprung disease. Some researchers argue that all familial Hirschsprung disease patients should be screened for the *RET* mutation responsible for MEN 2A because early diagnosis and thyroidectomy alters the disease course. Shah–Waardenburg consists of pigmentary anomalies (white forelock, iris hypoplasia, and patchy hypopigmentation). When central hypoventilation syndrome, also known as Ondine's curse, is associated with Hirschsprung disease, it is known as Haddad syndrome.
- Hirschsprung disease is occasionally associated with Bardet–Biedl syndrome (pigmentary retinopathy, obesity, hypogenitalism, mild mental retardation, and postaxial polydactyly).
- There are case reports of Di George, Silver–Russell, CHARGE, or Dandy–Walker syndrome associated with Hirschsprung disease, but these are not common associations.
- No cases of Kabuki syndrome have been reported in association with Hirschsprung disease.

Which gene(s) have been implicated in the autosomal dominant inheritance of Hirschsprung disease?

A. RET

B. EDNRB

C. SOX10

D. NTN

E. All of the above

LEARNING POINTS

- All of the above genes have been reported in an autosomal dominant pattern of inheritance (Amiel et al., 2008). However, they show incomplete penetrance and therefore carriers may not manifest Hirschsprung disease. The penetrance of the *RET* gene is greater in males than in females, which explains why inheritance of Hirschsprung disease is sex modified. It is also thought that there are modifying genes affecting the expression of implicated genes. Genetic interactions have been described between *EDNRB* and *RET* in the Mennonite population, where the incidence of Hirschsprung disease is 1 in 500. This has also been seen in South African studies where significant *EDNRB* and *RET* mutations in three kindreds were associated with increased penetrance in succeeding generations (Moore and Zaahl, 2015).
- The poor correlation between genotype and phenotype means that there is little benefit in screening for mutations. One exception (as previously mentioned) involves the particular mutations in the *RET* gene (affecting exons 10 and 11) that are associated with the cancer predisposition syndrome MEN 2A.
- Recent research has found variants in genes coding for semaphorins (proteins that guide developing nerve cells towards their final target) that, when associated with a *RET* mutation, can lead to Hirschsprung disease (Qian et al., 2015).

REFERENCES

Amiel J et al. Hirschsprung disease, associated syndromes and genetics: A review. *J Med Genet* 2008; 45: 1–14.

Moore SW, Zaahl M. Clinical and genetic correlations of familial Hirschsprung's disease. *J Pediatr Surg* 2015; 50: 285–288.

Qian et al. Functional loss of semaphorin 3C and/or semaphorin 3D and their epistatic interaction with Ret are critical to Hirschsprung disease liability. *Am J Human Genet* 2015; 96(4): 581.

ANSWERS

34.1	B
34.2	C
34.3	A
34.4	E

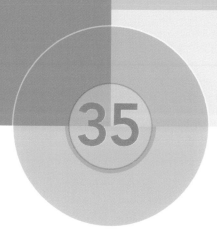
Radiology of a newborn with distal bowel obstruction: Case study

REVIEW 35.1 MULTIPLE CHOICE QUESTION

In the evaluation of a newborn infant with the plain abdominal radiograph shown, suggesting distal bowel obstruction (multiple dilated air-filled loops of the bowel), what is the preferred contrast agent when performing a diagnostic enema?

A. Near iso-osmolal water-soluble contrast
B. Barium
C. Hypo-osmolal water-soluble contrast
D. Saline
E. Hyper-osmolal water-soluble contrast

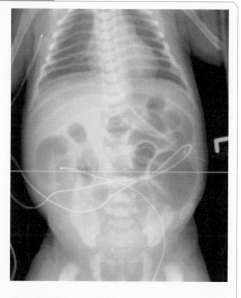

Figure 35.1 Plain abdominal x-ray.

LEARNING POINTS

1. Near iso-osmolal contrast is the preferred initial contrast in infants with a presumptive diagnosis of distal bowel obstruction. The main differential diagnoses include:
   a. Hirschsprung disease
   b. Neonatal small left colon
   c. Ileal atresia
   d. Meconium ileus
   e. Meconium plug syndrome
      i. Meconium plug syndrome and meconium ileus are potentially treatable disorders with a water-soluble contrast enema.
      ii. Barium offers no benefit in the initial diagnostic evaluation of distal bowel obstruction and can lead to further complications in the setting of perforation.
      iii. Hyper-osmolal agents such as Gastrograffin (1900 mOsm/L) should be avoided due to the massive fluid shifts, electrolyte imbalance, bowel necrosis (polysorbate component), and increased bowel distention in Hirschsprung disease.

2. The radiologic diagnosis of Hirschsprung disease is made with a contrast enema and the identification of a transition zone.
   a. A small-caliber catheter is placed in the rectum as close to the external sphincter as possible.
   b. Water-soluble contrast is introduced (iso-osmolal agents are preferred in neonates) in a controlled fashion under gravity.
   c. The critical imaging in Hirschsprung disease is the *initial lateral view* as contrast enters the colon.
   d. The aganglionic colon is often normal in caliber with an abrupt transition to the dilated proximal colon.
   e. The aganglionic segment is typically serrated in appearance due to aperistaltic contractions.
   f. An abnormal rectosigmoid ratio (<0.9) is often encountered in short segment Hirschsprung disease, but may be misleading in more extensive aganglionosis.
   g. The contrast enema is terminated when a zone of transition is identified.
   h. The radiographic diagnosis of total colonic aganglionosis may be difficult given that the colon may have a normal appearance, pseudo-transition zone, or microcolon.

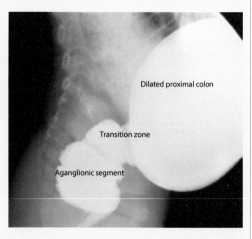

Dilated proximal colon

Transition zone

Aganglionic segment

Figure 35.2 Contrast enema.

ANSWER

35.1   A

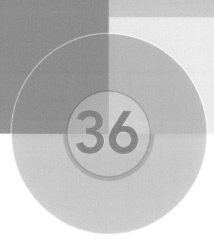

Pathology—Patient with possible Hirschsprung disease: Case study

36

A 3-year-old boy with a history of chronic constipation poor growth, and chronic abdominal distention is assessed in the outpatient clinic. You decide that Hirschsprung disease (HD) is on the differential diagnosis and perform a rectal biopsy.

REVIEW 36.1 MULTIPLE CHOICE QUESTION

The pathology report shows ganglion cells and hypertrophic nerves measuring 90 μm.

How will you proceed?

A. Proceed to a pull-through procedure.
B. Repeat the rectal biopsy as the biopsy was taken too low (below the dentate line).
C. Continue to treat the constipation.

REVIEW 36.2 MULTIPLE CHOICE QUESTION

The pathology report shows squamous epithelial cells and the absence of ganglion cells. No hypertrophic nerves are seen.

How will you proceed?

A. Proceed to a pull-through procedure.
B. Repeat the rectal biopsy as the biopsy was taken too low (below the dentate line).
C. Continue to treat the constipation.

HD is a congenital condition leading to a lack of ganglion cells in the seromuscular layer (Auerbach plexus) and the submucosa (Meissner plexus) of the bowel. The disease most commonly affects the distal large colon (short segment), but long segment disease, total colonic aganglionosis, and total intestinal aganglionosis also occur.

- Rectosigmoid 75%–80% of cases
- Splenic flexure or more proximal 10% of cases
- Total colonic aganglionosis: 5% (entire colon + rarely small bowel)

HD can also occur in combination with other conditions including:

- Down's syndrome (HD affects 10% of those with trisomy 21)
- Waardenburg syndrome
- Mowat–Wilson
- Congenital hypoventilation syndrome

The pathogenesis of HD is not fully understood, but the most popular hypotheses include:

- A disorder of target cell migration from the neural crest during embryonic development
- The degeneration of ganglion cells during development
- Abnormal differentiation of cells in an altered microenvironment

HD in most cases is not a genetic disease; however, numerous genes have been identified and are thought to be associated with the disease. These include:

- *RET*
- *EDNRB*
- *EDN3*

RET is a gene involved in the production of a protein required for cell signaling. Mutations within this gene leads to an abnormal RET protein that cannot transmit signals within the cell. Without RET protein signaling, enteric nerves do not function/develop properly, leading to HD.

EDNRB is a gene that provides instructions for the production of the protein called endothelin receptor type B. When this protein interacts with other proteins called endothelins, it transmits information from outside to inside the cell.

EDN3 is a gene that provides instructions for the protein endothelin 3, which interacts with endothelin receptor B. Together, they play an important role in the formation of enteric nerves.

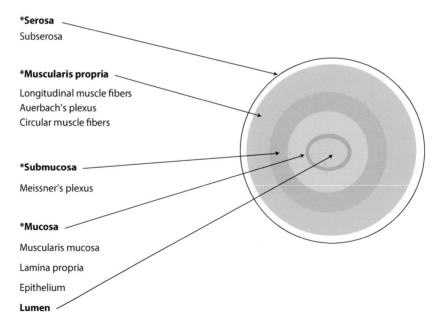

Figure 36.1 Bowel layers.

DIAGNOSIS

There are several methods used (often in combination) to diagnose HD and these include:

- Contrast enema
- Suction rectal biopsy
- Anorectal manometry

The contrast enema can be helpful in the diagnosis of HD if a transition zone is demonstrated, but its sensitivity is only about 80%. The contrast study is therefore used in combination with a rectal biopsy in most institutions, which has been reported to have >95% diagnostic accuracy.

Anorectal manometry is used sometimes to diagnose HD; however, its use is limited to children over the age of 12 months. One of the characteristics of HD is thought to be the fact that patients are unable to relax the internal anal sphincter in response to rectal distention, and this is the basis for the diagnosis of HD with anorectal manometry.

REVIEW 36.3 MULTIPLE CHOICE QUESTION

What is the characteristic finding on anorectal manometry for HD?

A. Presence of the rectoanal inhibitory reflex
B. Absence of the rectoanal inhibitory reflex

HISTOPATHOLOGY AND HD

The diagnostic accuracy of the rectal biopsy depends on a number of key factors:

- Site of the biopsy
- Representative sample of bowel being biopsied (i.e., taken from >1 cm above the dentate line)
- Adequate biopsy specimen
- Technical skills in processing of the specimen
- Correct interpretation by the pathologist
- Accurate reporting by the pathologist and subsequent interpretation by the operative surgeon

The basic criteria for the pathological diagnosis of HD are:

- Lack of ganglion cells in the submucosal ± the intramuscular nerve plexus of the intestinal wall
- Presence of hypertrophied nerve fibers and trunks

RECTAL BIOPSIES

- Suction rectal biopsy is recommended as the gold standard.
  - Suction rectal biopsies are more difficult to interpret than transmural biopsies because they only include the surface submucosal (Meissner) nerve plexus and do not contain the more richly ganglionated myenteric (Auerbach's) plexus.

- Transmural biopsies are, however, associated with a higher complication rate.
- Transmural (full-thickness) biopsy is recommended if more than one suction rectal biopsy has been inadequate for diagnosis. Transmural biopsies contain both plexuses; however, they can still be difficult to interpret if the tissue is poorly prepared.
- The biopsy must be taken *at least 1 cm* above the dentate line. Below this line is a recognized area of normal aganglionosis.
  - If tissue is taken from this "normal aganglionic" area, the histopathologist should identify epithelium that is different from that seen in the large intestine (squamous epithelial cells vs. columnar epithelial cells).
  - Care must be taken in the reporting of such findings to ensure that the surgeon does not misinterpret the biopsy as being consistent with HD.

FROZEN SECTION: WARNING!

- Frozen sections *are not recommended* in the primary diagnosis of HD.
  - It is only possible to get one to two slices on frozen section specimens, and *this is inadequate.*
- Frozen section can be extremely useful (in certain situations) for the surgeon to gain real-time information intra-operatively about surgical specimens (e.g., tumors).
- The surgeon relies on the pathologist to identify the transition zone and the normal bowel. The evaluation of the mucosal tissue and the transition zone for ganglion cells, however, is recognized to be difficult, and this is even more problematic in frozen section analysis.
- The guidelines state that 50–100 levels should be examined for each rectal biopsy tissue specimen, stained with hematoxylin and eosin (H + E).

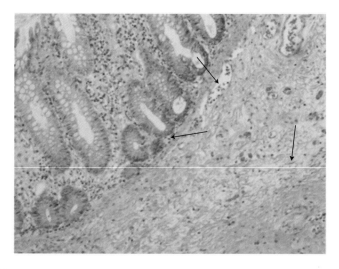

Figure 36.2 Hematoxylin and eosin stain (100×). Formalin fixation and hematoxylin and eosin-stained section. Normal ganglion cells within the submucosa as shown. No evidence of hypertrophied, tortuous, or increased nerves in submucosa.

HISTOPATHOLOGICAL PROCESSING

H + E stain:

- One of the principal stains in histology.
- Staining involves the application of hemalum, a complex formed from aluminum ions and hematein (an oxidation product of hematoxylin).
- Hemalum stains nuclei blue.
- The nuclear stain is followed by counterstaining with eosin, which colors other structures red/pink/orange.
- H + E staining remains the method of choice for the identification of ganglion cells.
- Regular biopsies for H + E slide studies require fixation of material in buffered formalin and then standard processing.

Regular biopsies for H + E slides require "only" fixation of material in buffered formalin and then standard processing, whereas application of additional histochemical staining for acetylcholinesterase (AChE) is associated with more complex processing; therefore, specimens should be sent to the pathology laboratory fresh without placing them in formalin.

Histochemical staining of frozen tissues for AChE demonstrates a larger mesh of thick, dense, and irregular nerve fibers.

- Formalin fixation and H + E stained (100×) section abnormal
- Note *no* ganglion cells within the submucosa
- Abundant thick (>40 μm), tortuous, and increased nerves in submucosa
- Hyperactivity of AChE becomes pathognomonic for HD.
- Histochemical staining (AChE) together with H + E staining was previously the gold standard in HD diagnosis.

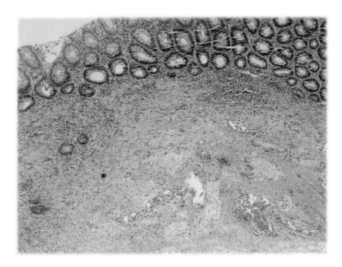

Figure 36.3 Hematoxylin + eosin stain. Formalin fixation and hematoxylin + eosin-stained section (50×) abnormal Note *no* ganglion cells within the submucosa Abundant thick (>40 μm), tortuous, and increased nerves in submucosa

147

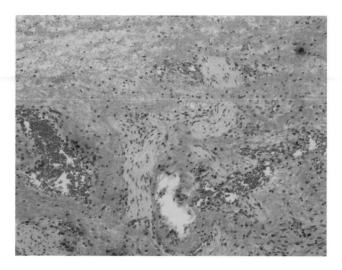

Figure 36.4 Pathology slide.

- Studies have demonstrated the high specificity of AChE staining, but with *inadequate* sensitivity of ~85%.
- False-negative results are mostly connected with:
  - Superficial biopsies (without muscularis mucosa)
  - Immaturity of the enzyme system (found in patients under the age of 2 years)
  - Technical variations in staining
  - Biopsies from premature infants

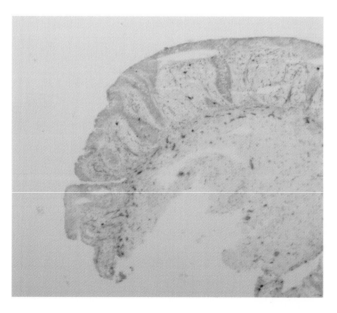

Figure 36.5 Acetylcholinesterase—suction rectal biopsy. Abnormal acetylcholinesterase-stained frozen tissue. Note thickened and increased nerve fibers within the lamina propria extending towards the surface (50×).

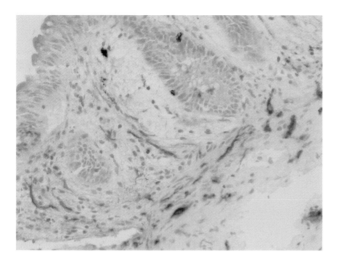

Figure 36.6 Abnormal acetylcholinesterase stained frozen tissue (200×).

Typical morphological AChE staining pictures characteristic of HD are detected only in the distal part of the large intestine (beneath the splenic flexure) because innervation of this intestinal section is different. Thus, diagnosis applying AChE staining of specimens taken from the ascending colon and transverse colon does not provide reliable information.

BIOPSIES

- If microscopic examination confirms the presence of ganglion cells, one can reject the diagnosis of HD.
  - If ganglion cells are not seen, further tests are required to prove HD.
  - The presence of thickened mucosal and submucosal nerve fibers (in the absence of ganglion cells) confirms HD on AChE staining.

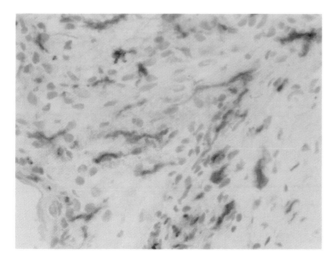

Figure 36.7 Abnormal acetylcholinesterase stained frozen tissue (400×).

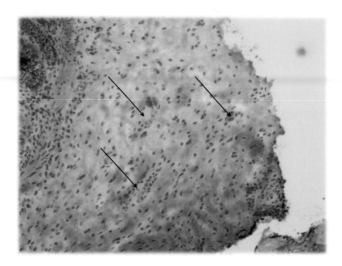

Figure 36.8 Diff-Quik (100×). Frozen preparation—intra-operative Diff-Quik-stained section normal. Note ganglion cells within the submucosa (arrows).

- However, if the characteristic findings on AChE staining are not met, clinicians should consider obtaining additional specimens and should observe the patient.
- If problems with the identification of ganglion cells occur in H + E slides, one has to perform additional immunohistochemical or histochemical tests (S100, NSE, and/or Diff-Quik).

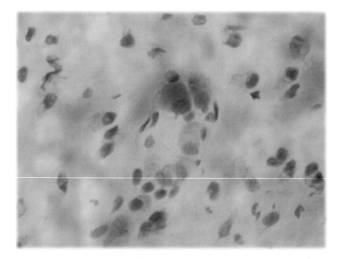

Figure 36.9 Diff-Quik (400×). Frozen preparation—intra-operative Diff-Quik-stained section normal. Ganglion cells show eccentric nucleus, plasmacytoid morphology, and amphophilic cytoplasm. Prominent nucleoli and bluish Nissl substance make it easy to identify. Diff-Quik stain is fast: frozen preparation, 90 seconds; hematoxylin and eosin stain, about 4 minutes.

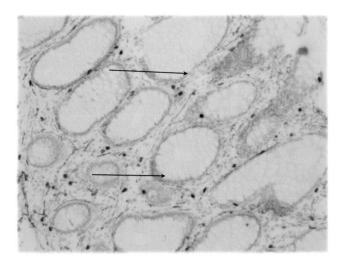

Figure 36.10 Calretinin stain (100×). Normal calretinin-stained section. Note slender neurites within the lamina propria (arrows).

Diff-Quik is a Romanowsky stain variant based on the Wright–Giemsa stain. The Diff-Quik stain consists of three solutions:

1. Diff-Quik fixative reagent: triarylmethane dye, methanol
2. Diff-Quik solution I (eosinophilic): xanthene dye, pH buffer, sodium azide
3. Diff-Quik solution II (basophilic): thiazide dye, pH buffer

In HD, calretinin immunohistochemistry can add diagnostic value to specimens with inadequate submucosa or rarely seen ganglion cells.

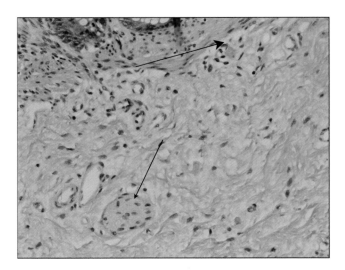

Figure 36.11 Hematoxylin and eosin (100×). Hematoxylin and eosin-stained section; transitional zone. Note *rare* ganglion cell (thick arrow). Thick (80-μm) nerve in submucosa (thin arrow).

- The presence of ganglion cells consistently correlates with calretinin-positive thin nerve fibrils (neurites) as shown in the image above.
- The calretinin-positive fibrils are absent in the aganglionic bowel.
- Faint positivity of the thick submucosal and subserosal nerves in the absence of ganglion cells and calretinin-positive nerve fibrils is characteristic of the transition zone (junction of aganglionic to normal bowel).

FURTHER READING

Barberi LEJ. Proposed recommendations and guidelines for diagnosis of Hirschsprung's disease in mucosal and submucosal biopsies from the rectum. *Rev Col Gastroenterol* 2011; 26(4): 274–279.

Fernandez RM et al. Pathways systematically associated to Hirschsprung's disease. *Orphanet J Rare Dis* 2013; 8: 187.

Łukasz S, Andrzej M. Diagnosis of Hirschsprung's disease with particular emphasis on histopathology. A systematic review of current literature. *Prz Gastroenterol* 2014; 9(5): 264–269.

Maia DM. The reliability of frozen-section diagnosis in the pathological evaluation of Hirschsprung's disease. *Am J Surg Path* 2000; 24(12): 1675–1677.

Miedema JR, Hunt HV. Practical issues for frozen section diagnosis in gastrointestinal and liver diseases. *J Gastrointestin Liver Dis* 2010; 19(2), 181–185.

Shayan K et al. Reliability of intraoperative frozen sections in the management of Hirschsprung's disease. *J Ped Surg* 2004; 39(9): 1345–1348.

ANSWERS

36.1   C
36.2   B
36.3   B

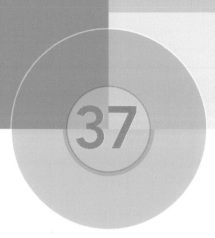

CASE HISTORY

- Below are radiographic images of a newborn infant with Hirschsprung disease.
- Consider the images below.

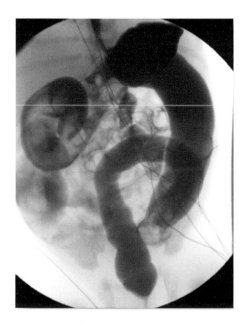

Figure 37.1 Contrast enema. How would you manage this patient?

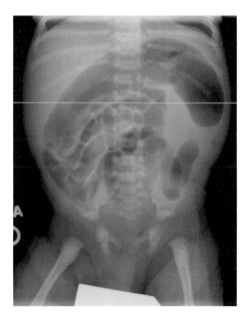

Figure 37.2 Plain radiograph. This infant was managed with rectal irrigations. The infant was clinically well. What is your opinion of the radiograph?

QUESTIONS

- How would you plan to perform the pull-through procedure, given the information provided?
- What do you need to consider?

This child was initially thought to have sigmoid disease based on the information provided by the contrast enema. The transition zone was thought to be in the sigmoid, and therefore the child's pull-through was approached transanally.

Ganglionic bowel however could not be identified through the transanal approach and therefore the procedure was converted to laparoscopic. The bowel could not be mobilized laparoscopically because of excessive bowel distension and hence the child required a laparotomy. Clearly a laparoscopy first with confirmation of the transition zone should have been the first step. This is an excellent example of why starting transanal only is a potential pitfall.

An indication that the transition may have been more proximal than previously suspected is suggested by the plain abdominal radiograph as the bowel is not being decompressed proximal to the splenic flexure, despite irrigations usually a sigmoid transition zone case easily decompresses with irrigations.

LEARNING POINTS

- This patient was found to have Hirschsprung disease proximal to the splenic flexure.
- Extensive colonic mobilization that *would not have* been possible through a transanal approach was required.
- This child had a long operative procedure that could have been avoided.

In hindsight, this patient should have had:
- Laparoscopic biopsies to map the bowel to aid in operative planning, and consideration for an ileostomy, and wait for permanent histology sections.

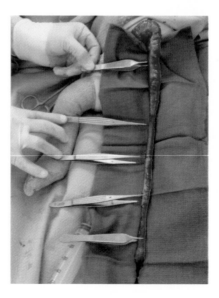

Figure 37.3 Laparotomy showing length of abnormal bowel.

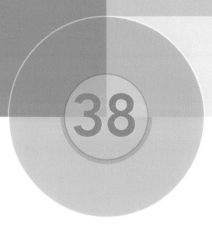

Total colonic Hirschsprung disease

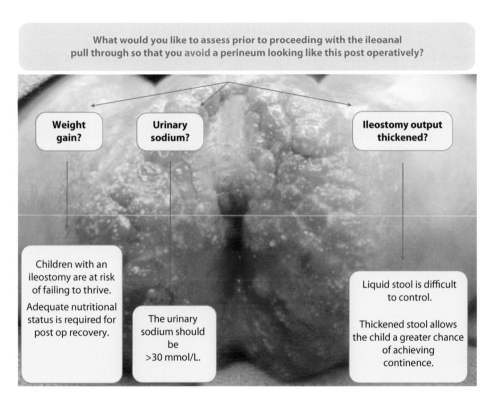

What would you like to assess prior to proceeding with the ileoanal pull through so that you avoid a perineum looking like this post operatively?

Weight gain?

Urinary sodium?

Ileostomy output thickened?

Children with an ileostomy are at risk of failing to thrive.

Adequate nutritional status is required for post op recovery.

The urinary sodium should be >30 mmol/L.

Liquid stool is difficult to control.

Thickened stool allows the child a greater chance of achieving continence.

Figure 38.1 Perineum of a patient that underwent an ileoanal pull-through too early in life.

Total colonic Hirschsprung disease: Case history

- 6 years old.
- Diagnosed with total colonic Hirschsprung disease at birth.
- He has an ileostomy that has previously been revised, with loss of 30 cm of small bowel.
- The family is keen to have an ileoanal pull-through and reverse the ileostomy.

LEARNING POINTS

- Total colonic Hirschsprung disease patients can be challenging to manage following an ileoanal or ileo-Duhamel pull-through. In our opinion, these children should be managed initially with an ileostomy, until they are at an age when the ileostomy output is thickened, and this can be with the aid of loperamide, water-soluble fiber, and constipating foods. The ideal timing for the pull-through is of 6 to 18 months of age.
- Very liquid small bowel contents on the perineum cause excoriation, which can be difficult to manage; however, with the continued introduction of very effective barrier creams/diaper rash creams, this is becoming easier to manage.
- If the parents are highly motivated and dedicated to meticulous skin care, the surgeon may consider performing the operation earlier in life, but the risks of perineal skin breakdown should not be underestimated.

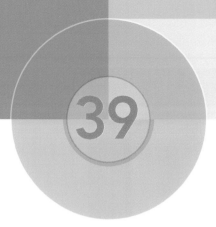
Transanal-only approach—Technical steps: Case study

CASE HISTORY

- A newborn male infant was diagnosed with Hirschsprung disease after presenting on day 6 of life with poor stooling, abdominal distention, and vomiting.
- He was managed with rectal irrigations, and irrigations were successful in decompressing him.
- His contrast enema is shown below.

REVIEW 39.1 MULTIPLE CHOICE QUESTION

Where is the transition zone?

A. Sigmoid
B. Splenic flexure
C. Transverse colon

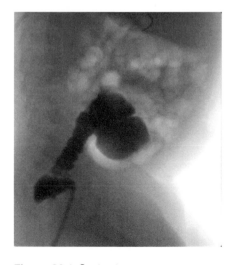

Figure 39.1 Contrast enema.

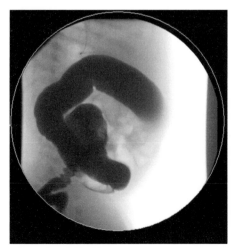

Figure 39.2 Contrast enema.

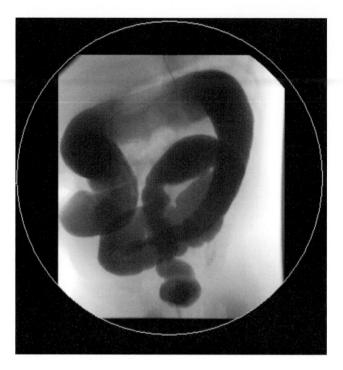

Figure 39.3 Contrast enema. Is a transanal only approach a consideration?

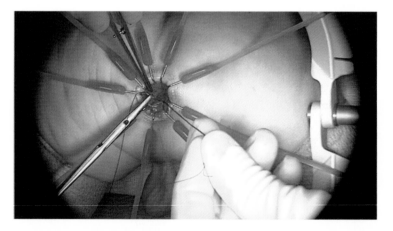

Figure 39.4 Transanal pull-through operative images. Sutures are inserted circumferentially 1 cm above the dentate line to mark the line of initial full-thickness dissection.

> ## LEARNING POINTS
>
> ■ The transition zone on the contrast enema is in the mid-sigmoid.
> ■ This case was suitable for a transanal-only procedure without the need for a colostomy.

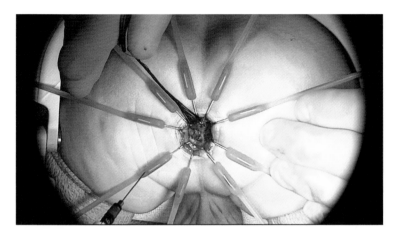

Figure 39.5 Full-thickness dissection in order to establish the Swenson plane.

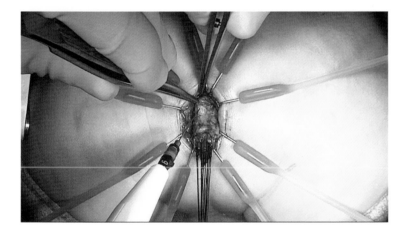

Figure 39.6 Swenson plane. Patient is in prone position.

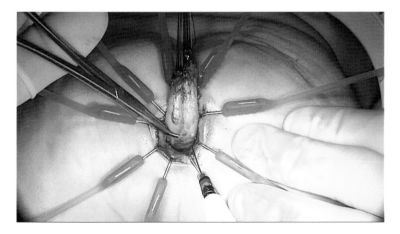

Figure 39.7 Peritoneal reflection.

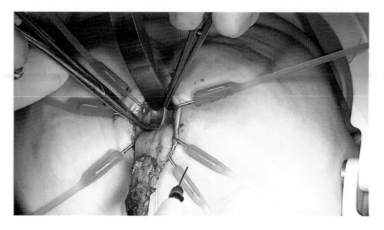

Figure 39.8 Posterior dissection.

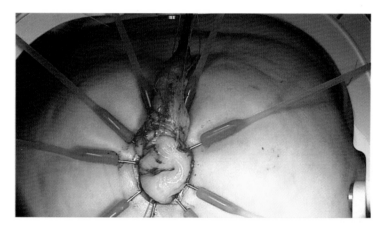

Figure 39.9 The anterior rectum frees up before the posterior, and thus the biopsy can be done in the sigmoid.

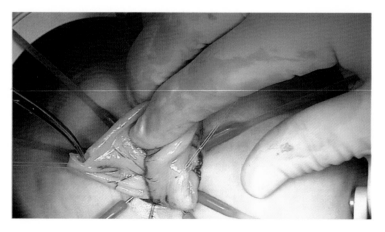

Figure 39.10 Full-thickness rectal biopsy.

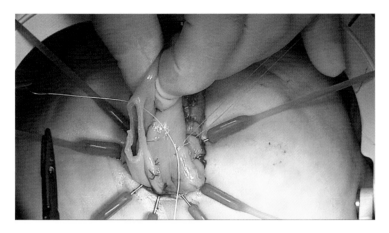

Figure 39.11 Biopsy site closed.

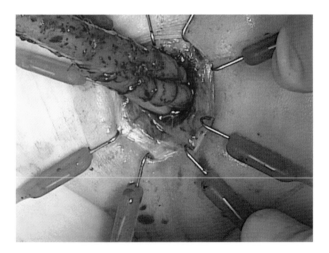

Figure 39.12 Further mobilization of the colon transanally.

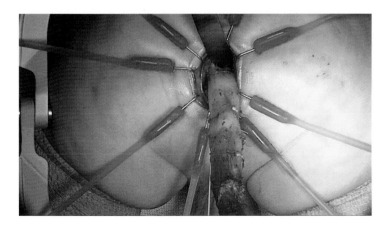

Figure 39.13 Sigmoid now fully mobilized.

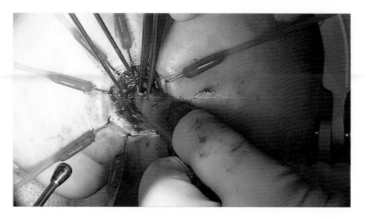

Figure 39.14 Site of normal ganglionic bowel identified. Bowel trimmed in preparation for anastomosis.

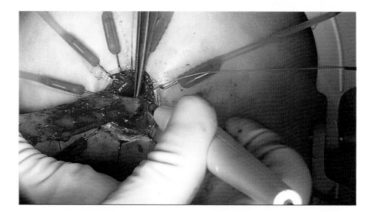

Figure 39.15 Start of anastomosis.

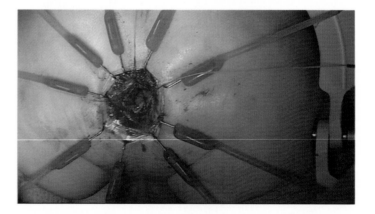

Figure 39.16 Circumferential anastomosis with preservation of the dentate line.

ANSWER

39.1   A

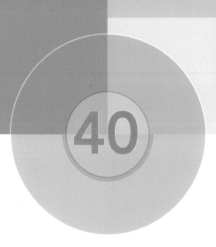

Pull-through procedure
for Hirschsprung disease:
Case study

40

CASE HISTORY

- This is the contrast enema (Figure 40.1) of a newborn infant with confirmed Hirschsprung disease on suction rectal biopsy.
- The child had been managed at home with rectal irrigations and had been clinically well.

REVIEW 40.1 MULTIPLE CHOICE QUESTION

Where is the transition zone?

A. Rectum
B. Total colonic
C. Splenic flexure
D. Hepatic flexure
E. Proximal sigmoid

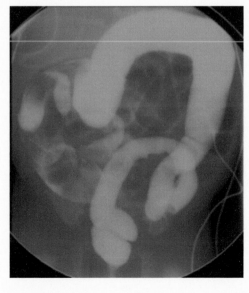

Figure 40.1 Contrast enema.

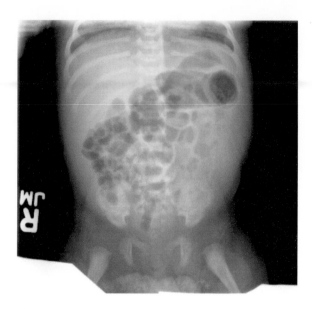

Figure 40.2 Plain radiograph following rectal irrigations. What is your interpretation of this radiograph? Are the irrigations working?

REVIEW 40.2 MULTIPLE CHOICE QUESTION

At the time of the elective laparoscopic pull-through procedure, turbid fluid was found in the right upper quadrant. The bowel was noted to be inflamed.

How would you proceed?

A. Cancel the operation and let inflammation improve with antibiotics
B. Perform a leveling colostomy
C. Perform an ileostomy with full-thickness colonic mapping
D. Perform an ileostomy

The abdominal x-ray shows that there appears to be some dilation of the transverse colon and incomplete decompression despite rectal irrigations.

At this point, the surgeons proceeded with a laparoscopic-assisted pull-through as the child was clinically well.

- Due to concern of turbid fluid, enterocolitis was suspected. Therefore,
  - The bowel was mapped with multiple full-thickness colonic biopsies in order to identify the normal ganglionated bowel and to aid in the preoperative planning for the definitive pull-through procedure. An ileostomy was performed.
  - The frozen section biopsies are shown in Table 40.1.

Table 40.1 Results of the intraoperative biopsies

Bowel segment	Histopathology
Rectum	No ganglion cells
Sigmoid	No ganglion cells
Descending colon	Acute mucosal inflammation with necrosis; full-thickness inflammation with necrosis of the muscular wall
Transverse colon	Ganglion cells present; multiple foci of acute inflammation
Ascending colon	Ganglion cells present; multiple foci of acute inflammation
Small bowel	No significant pathological alteration; ganglion cells present

The patient was managed with an **ileostomy** at this time.

LEARNING POINTS

- This child was at home and the parents were performing the rectal irrigations after formal training in the hospital.
- However, at the time of the elective pull-through procedure, this infant has evidence of subclinical enterocolitis. This was confirmed on the histopathology of the colonic mapping biopsies.
- With these pathology findings and those observed at laparoscopy, the safest surgical approach is to perform an ileostomy and to thereby defunctionalize the bowel.

How would you proceed following formation of the ileostomy?

- The child subsequently underwent a pull-through procedure and the transition zone was found to be in the descending colon.

ANSWERS

40.1   E
40.2   C

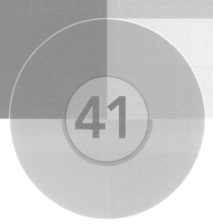

Examination of a Hirschsprung patient: Case study

41

CASE HISTORY

- You are referred a patient with Hirschsprung disease who underwent a pull-through as a baby, who is not doing well with potty training.
- She is now 5 years old and continues to have problems with daily soiling.
- The parents tell you that she had a Soave pull-through as an infant and there were no complications following surgery.
- She is currently not on any laxatives or stool softeners.
- You perform an examination under anesthesia to assess the anatomy and your findings are shown in Figure 41.1.

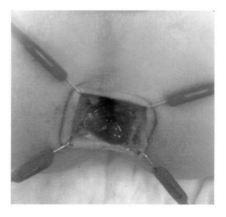

Figure 41.1 Examination of the anal canal. What do you notice on examination under anaesthesia?

The exam reveled a damaged dentate line at the 4 o'clock to 8 o'clock position, which makes you conclude that there is a reduced likelihood that this child that will achieve future continence.

The contrast enema Figure 41.2 shows widening of the pre-sacral space, suggestive of a Soave cuff, which can physiologically obstruct the pull-through.

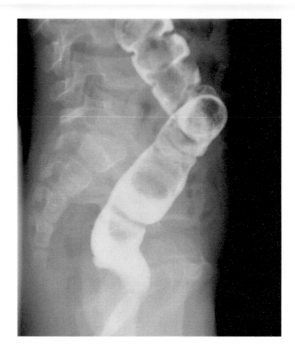

Figure 41.2 Lateral image of contrast enema.

LEARNING POINTS

- Patients with Hirschsprung disease who are "not doing well" postoperatively need to be thoroughly assessed.
- This evaluation entails an **EUA** to check the dentate line, repeat **rectal biopsy** to check the pathology, and a **contrast enema**.
- This patient due to the loss of the dentate line needs a bowel management program with daily enemas for now. Their sphincters may be adequate to gain them bowel control in the long run. If there is a soave cuff that is obstructing it may need to be removed via a redo procedure.

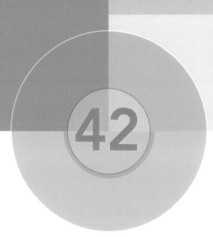

Obstructive symptoms in a Hirschsprung patient: Case study

42

- This patient was diagnosed with Hirschsprung disease as a newborn infant.
- She underwent a laparoscopic-assisted transanal Soave pull-through.
- She did well following the pull-through; however, she has been experiencing problems with constipation for several years, despite medical therapy (senna 60 mg and stool softeners).
- More recently, she has been having episodes of enterocolitis requiring hospital admissions, and she is currently taking prophylactic antibiotics to reduce these episodes.
- Multiple attempts have been made to improve her stooling with Botox injections, which have failed.

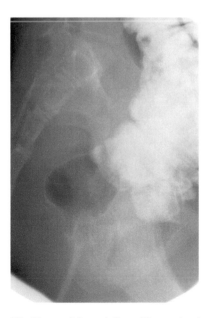

Figure 42.1 Contrast enema. What is your interpretation of the contrast enema?

LEARNING POINTS

- The obstructive symptoms that this child has been experiencing after initially doing well post-Soave pull-through are characteristic of a Soave cuff causing a degree of obstruction.
- On the contrast study, there is widening of the pre-sacral space, which is characteristic of a Soave cuff.
- The surgeon did not appreciate that a cuff was the problem, believing that hypertonic sphincter was the cause of the obstructive symptoms, and has tried repeated injections with Botox.
- This child should also undergo an examination under anesthesia and rectal biopsy to confirm the diagnosis of a cuff by digital exam and exclude a transition zone pull-through. The cuff is palpable on rectal examination (usually felt as a rubbery ring outside of the pull-through).
- She ultimately required a redo pull-through procedure to resect the Soave cuff. This was possible transanally and the operative images are shown below.

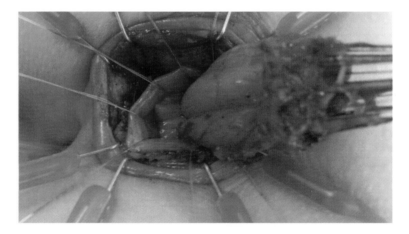

Figure 42.2 Intraoperative image. Soave cuff identified and removed. Pull-through then resutured in place. Postoperatively obstructive symptoms resolved.

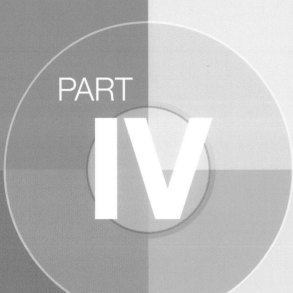

INVESTIGATION ALGORITHM

PROBLEMATIC PATIENT POST-PULL-THROUGH

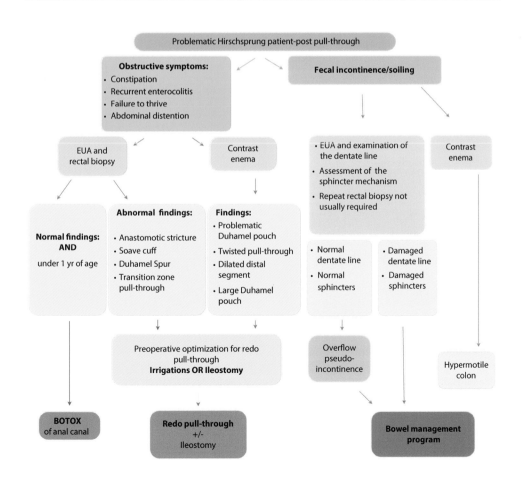

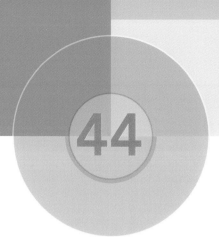

Problematic pull-through—Postoperative enterocolitis: Case study

CASE HISTORY

- A 3-month-old male infant with Hirschsprung disease underwent a Swenson transanal pull-through in the newborn period.
- He developed enterocolitis postoperatively requiring hospitalization.
- **How are you going to assess this patient?**

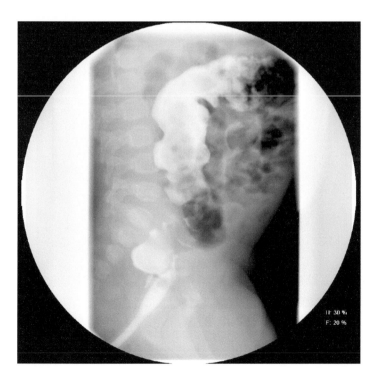

Figure 44.1 Contrast enema. What is your opinion of the contrast enema?

EXAMINATION UNDER ANESTHESIA

- **Severe anal stricture.**
- Repeat rectal biopsy not performed on this occasion as the pull-through needs to be redone, and the histology can be rechecked at that time. Also it would have been technically very difficult to biopsy proximal to the stricture.

LEARNING POINTS

- The problematic patient post-pull-through procedure should be worked up systematically to exclude all potential reasons that the child may not be emptying well.
- Contrast enema
- Examination under anesthesia (EUA)
- Rectal biopsy

The pre-sacral space is normal on the lateral image. Irregularity of the distal colon suggest enterocolitis. This distal area appears narrow, with proximal dilatation suggestive of a stricture.

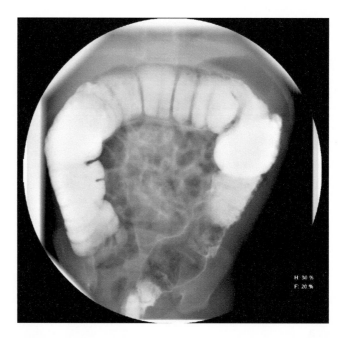

Figure 44.2 Contrast enema showing narrowing of the distal segment, proximal dilatation, and irregularity of the left colon wall consistent with enterocolitis.

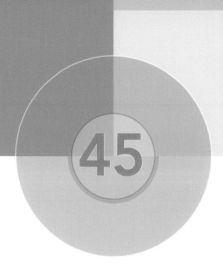

Problematic pull-through— A patient who originally presented with cecal perforation: Case study

45

- A 2-year-old boy with Down's syndrome and Hirschsprung disease (HD) presents to your outpatient clinic for ongoing surgical care.
- He was diagnosed in the newborn period with HD after developing a cecal perforation in the first week of life.

REVIEW 45.1 MULTIPLE CHOICE QUESTION

What level is the transition zone most likely to be considering the history of a cecal perforation?

A. Total colonic disease
B. Ascending colon
C. Transverse colon
D. Splenic flexure
E. Rectosigmoid
F. Descending colon

He was managed at this time with an ileostomy, and leveling biopsies were performed showing transition zone at the hepatic flexure. He ultimately underwent pull-through of the right colon.

REVIEW 45.2 MULTIPLE CHOICE QUESTION

After his pull-through he had severe failure to thrive due to the recurrent episodes of enterocolitis.

How are you going to manage this patient?

A. Bowel management with rectal enemas
B. High-dose laxatives
C. Ileostomy
D. Colostomy

REVIEW 45.3 MULTIPLE CHOICE QUESTION

He attends your clinic for follow-up. He is now doing well with his ileostomy.

What is your interpretation of the contrast enema?

A. Normal
B. Stricture
C. Duhamel pull-through

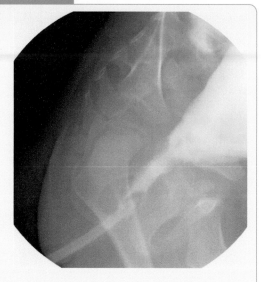

Figure 45.1 Contrast enema, lateral view.

LEARNING POINTS

- The stricture is probably due to ischemia in the pulled-through bowel secondary to the original division of the middle colic vessels.
- This child was failing to thrive and was therefore managed with an ileostomy. An ileostomy was chosen so that the remaining colon could be used for the redo pull-through.

ANSWERS

45.1	B
45.2	C
45.3	B

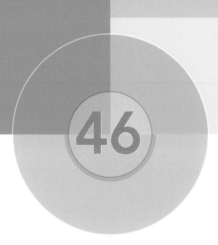
Recurrent Hirschsprung-associated enterocolitis: Case study

CASE HISTORY

- A 2-year-old male infant was diagnosed with Hirschsprung disease in the newborn period.
- A transanal Soave pull-through was performed at 3 months of age.
- The child presented for evaluation following recurrent episodes of Hirschsprung-associated enterocolitis (HAEC) at the age of 18 months.

REVIEW 46.1 MULTIPLE CHOICE QUESTION

What could be the cause of the recurrent HAEC?

A. Soave cuff

B. Stricture

C. Transition zone pull-through

D. All of the above

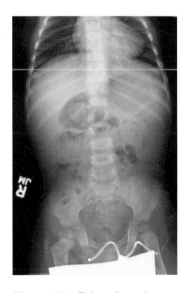

Figure 46.1 Plain radiograph. What is your interpretation of this X-ray? What is your next step in this patient's management?

EXAMINATION UNDER ANESTHESIA OF THE ANUS

On digital examination, the boy was found to have a circumferential rubbery ring along the hollow of the sacrum consistent with a Soave cuff.

The abdominal x-ray shows an impacted colon, full of formed stool.

MANAGEMENT

- Redo pull-through procedure.
- Soave cuff removed.
- Histopathology confirmed there to be normal ganglionated bowel with no hypertrophied nerves.

After his redo procedure, he continued to have occasional HAEC despite reconfirmed normal anatomy and no stricture but with much less frequency from previous.

What else could be wrong? What other management strategies are available to you?

LEARNING POINTS

- This patient was managed with Botox injection into the external sphincter to help reduce anal spasms, which are thought to contribute to failure to evacuate stool in those under 2 years of age.
- After one year no further episodes of HAEC occurred.

ANSWER

46.1   D

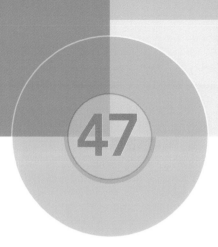

Problematic postoperative Hirschsprung patient: Case study

47

- This is the plain x-ray of a 2-year-old girl with total colonic Hirschsprung disease and she has had a pull-through procedure performed at 12 months of age.
- She is currently having difficulties with constipation and postoperatively has had episodes of enterocolitis.

REVIEW 47.1 MULTIPLE CHOICE QUESTION

Which technique was used for the original pull-through?

A. Soave
B. Swenson
C. Duhamel

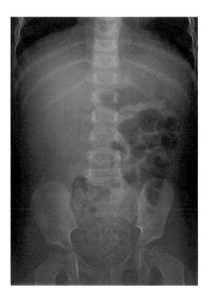

Figure 47.1 Plain abdominal radiograph. How are you going to manage this patient?

REVIEW 47.2 MULTIPLE CHOICE QUESTION

This is the contrast enema showing the post-Duhamel pull-through. What does this contrast enema show?

A. Soave cuff
B. Normal
C. Duhamel spur
D. Stricture

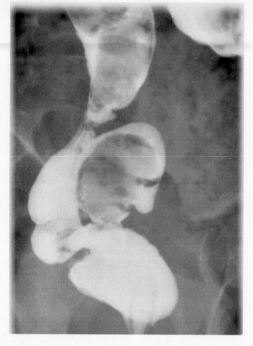

Figure 47.2 Contrast enema.

Due to recurrent episodes of recurrent enterocolotis the decision was made to perform a redo of the pull-through. Resection of the spur as a first step was another option.

DUHAMEL PULL-THROUGH

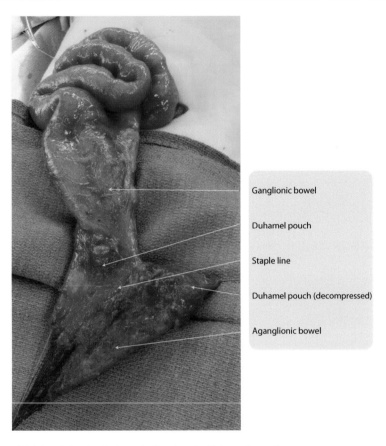

Ganglionic bowel

Duhamel pouch

Staple line

Duhamel pouch (decompressed)

Aganglionic bowel

Figure 47.3 Mobilized distal pull-through showing the Duhamel pouch.

LEARNING POINTS

- Staple lines in the pelvis in a child with a history of Hirschsprung disease on abdominal x-ray would suggest that the original procedure was a Duhamel pull-through.
- There is marked fecal loading in the Duhamel pouch, which is failing to empty.
- In children with a Duhamel pull-through, it is important to exclude a Duhamel spur.
- Excision of the spur with stapler or removal of the pouch and conversion to an ileoanal pull-through are two options for treatment. In this case due to significant symptoms of failure to thrive and her very young age a more definitive redo procedure was chosen.

ANSWERS

47.1   C

47.2   C

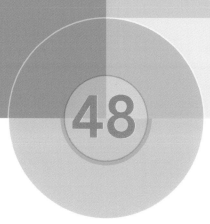

Redo surgery for Hirschsprung disease: Case study

48

CASE HISTORY

- This 5-year-old child has had a previous pull-through procedure and presents with a history of constipation and soiling. There are regular episodes of distension and since surgery have been three episodes of enterocolitis.
- Botox of the anal canal has been done several times with no improvement.

What does the contrast enema show?

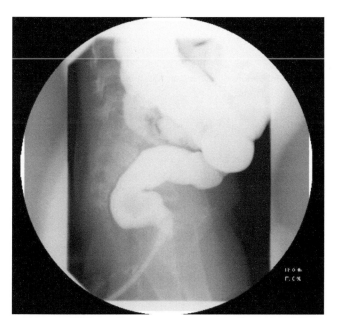

Figure 48.1 Contrast enema. Normal. No evidence of a Soave cuff.

REVIEW 48.1 MULTIPLE CHOICE QUESTION

How are you going to evaluate/treat this patient?

A. Check the original pathology report
B. Maximize medical therapy for constipation
C. Cecostomy/antegrade continence enema (ACE)
D. Examination under anesthesia, repeat rectal biopsy

EUA

Partially lost dentate line

REVIEW 48.2 MULTIPLE CHOICE QUESTION

The histopathologist states that the biopsy demonstrates a transition zone. Which of these reports is in keeping with a transition zone pull-through?

A. Ganglion cells present and no hypertrophied nerves seen
B. Ganglion cells present and nerve fibers of 70 μm seen
C. Ganglion cells seen and nerve fibers of 25 μm seen
D. Ganglion cells seen and nerve fibers of 40 μm seen
E. Answers B, C, and D

LEARNING POINTS

- The histopathologist must report on the presence or absence of ganglion cells and on the size of the nerve fibers seen. Nerve fibers of 40 μm or less are considered normal.

MANAGEMENT

- This child requires a redo procedure for a retained transition zone and obstructive symptoms. The redo of the pull-through needs to reach to healthy colon with both normal ganglion cells and normal size nerves. This redo is needed, given his significant obstructive symptoms.
- The additional concern in this child, however, is the damage to the dentate line, which is likely to impair his potential for future fecal continence, and he may require a cecostomy/ACE/Malone to be socially clean.

ANSWERS

48.1   D
48.2   B

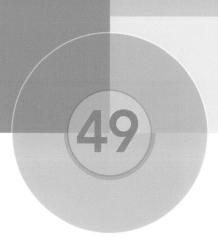

Enterocolitis after a Hirschsprung pull-through: Case study

49

- This patient was diagnosed with Hirschsprung disease when he was a few days old and underwent a Soave endorectal pull-through with laparoscopy as a newborn infant.
- Since the time of the pull-through, he has had many episodes of enterocolitis.

He presents with distension and fever. The radiograph demonstrates significant colonic dilatation. He is now 2 years of age. This child requires colonic decompression with rectal irrigations and antibiotics, with adequate intravenous fluid replacement. He recovers and you perform a contrast enema.

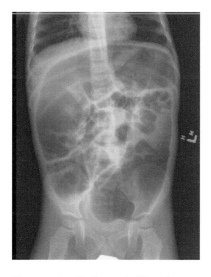

Figure 49.1 Radiograph. What does this radiograph show? How would you manage this child?

REVIEW 49.1 MULTIPLE CHOICE QUESTION

What are the most likely explanations for this child presenting with enterocolitis following successful pull-through surgery at the age of 2 years?

A. Transition zone pull-through
B. Viral gastroenteritis
C. Retained Soave cuff/anastomotic stricture
D. Damage to the dentate line
E. Answers A, C, and D
F. Answers A and C

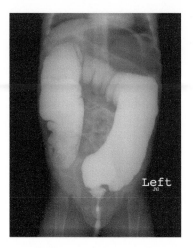

Figure 49.2 Contrast enema at the age of 2 years. What information does the contrast enema give you?

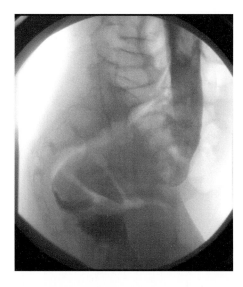

Figure 49.3 Lateral image.

There is narrowing of the bowel distally with colonic distention more proximally, which is suggestive of a stricture.

The lateral image does not reveal widening of the pre-sacral space, so a Soave cuff is unlikely to be the cause of the obstructive symptoms.

This child needs a redo of his pull-through to manage the stricture.

ANSWER

49.1   F

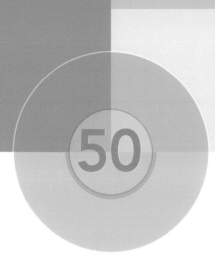

Six-year-old boy with known Hirschsprung's, trisomy 21, and obstructive symptoms: Case study

50

CASE HISTORY

- This is the case of a 6-year-old boy with known Hirschsprung disease (HD) and trisomy 21. He had a pull-through procedure as a newborn infant and the family have come to you for a second opinion.
- The child describes obstructive symptoms. He has a long-standing history of abdominal distension and episodes of fecal incontinence, usually at night time, and on occasion passes large stools. He has had one episode of Hirschsprung-associated enterocolitis in the previous 12 months requiring hospitalization.
- His weight gain is suboptimal and his appetite is poor.

Which pull-through procedure is he most likely to have had, given the clinical information and contrast enema images you have been provided with?

How are you going to manage this child?

What investigations would you like to perform in addition to the contrast enema?

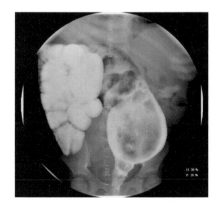

Figure 50.1 Contrast enema. What is your interpretation of the contrast enema?

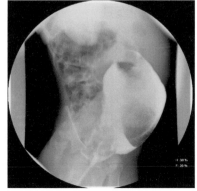

Figure 50.2 Contrast enema.

A Soave pull-through is the most likely previous procedure. The contrast enema shows the distal colon to be narrow and potentially externally constricted in the very terminal portion. This is most commonly secondary to a retained Soave cuff or could be due to a stricture. On the lateral image, there is excessive space between the concavity of the sacrum and the distal pull-through consistent with a retained Soave cuff.

This child requires further management. He is describing obstructive symptoms and has had episodes of enterocolitis. His weight gain is suboptimal and his appetite is poor, and nutrition input is important.

This child requires evaluation in the operating room. He requires an examination under anesthesia of the anus to:

- Assess the dentate line—is it intact? Will it help to contribute to continence?
- Assess for a retained Soave cuff
- Assess for an anastomotic stricture
- Perform a repeat rectal biopsy to ensure this is not a transition pull-through

Repeat rectal biopsy

No ganglion cells
No hypertrophied nerves

What conclusion do you draw from this biopsy result?

How are you going to manage this patient?

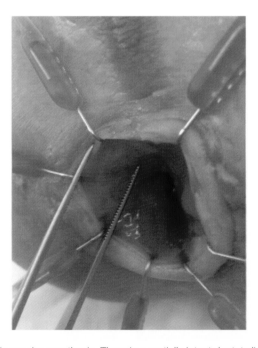

Figure 50.3 Examination under anesthesia. There is a partially intact dentate line as indicated by the forceps. The dentate line is absent at the 6 o'clock position. This amount of dentate line should be enough to allow for normal anal canal sensation.

LEARNING POINTS

Points for consideration:

1. This child has trisomy 21 and associated developmental delay.
2. His potential for bowel control and toilet training is compromised by his Down syndrome, but also due to partial loss of the dentate line.

REVIEW 50.1 MULTIPLE CHOICE QUESTION

Does he require a redo procedure in your opinion?

A. Yes
B. No

LEARNING POINTS

- We believe that this child should undergo a redo procedure. There are a number of ways that this child could be managed and these should be discussed with the parents.
- In this case, the child has been found to have had a previous transition zone pull-through, which is likely to be the cause of his obstructive symptoms. A retained Soave cuff may also be contributing. This is coupled with the fact that his dentate line has been partially lost, which will impair his continence potential, in addition to his underlying Down's syndrome.

The options for his management therefore must take these factors into account.

Obstructive symptom management of soiling

The options for his management are

1. Rectal irrigations (but this may be challenging for the parents, given his age) and redo surgery in the future ± covering/defunctioning ileostomy.
2. Temporary ileostomy in order for him to gain weight and thrive with a view to redo surgery in the future with an appendicostomy.
3. Perform redo surgery only ± ileostomy.
4. Permanent colostomy (with modern bowel management techniques, a permanent colostomy can be avoided in virtually all cases).
5. Rectal irrigations, redo pull-through with temporary defunctioning ileostomy, and an appendicostomy.

The surgeon must consider the child's potential for continence. As mentioned, his dentate line is damaged, so he may require additional bowel management strategies in order for him to be kept clean.

Which of the above options would you choose?

LEARNING POINTS

- We managed this child with Option 5.

ANSWER

50.1 A

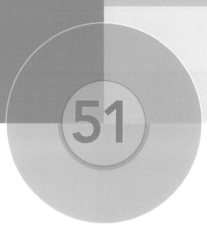

Two-year-old child with known Hirschsprung's, now with failure to thrive: Case study

51

CASE HISTORY

- This is the case of a child with known Hirschsprung disease who underwent an ileo-anal Duhamel pull-through in the newborn period.
- The child is now 2 years old and is failing to thrive (5th centile for weight) and is having difficulty stooling, chronic abdominal distension, and has developed Hirschsprung-associated enterocolitis.
- Multiple Botox injections have been performed in the past without improvement.

REVIEW 51.1 MULTIPLE CHOICE QUESTION

How are you going to assess/manage this patient?

A. Start stimulant laxatives (e.g., senna) and review in 4 weeks in the outpatient clinic with a plain abdominal radiograph.

B. Perform an examination under anesthesia to establish whether there is an anatomical problem.

C. Inject Botox into the anal sphincters.

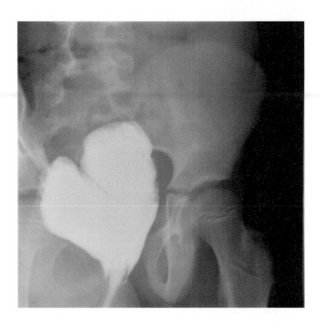

Figure 51.1 Contrast enema. Contrast enema is seen to enter the Duhamel pouch.

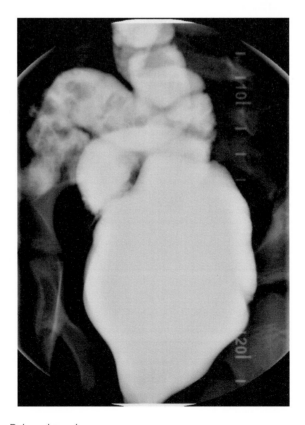

Figure 51.2 Mega Duhamel pouch.

As per the clinical protocol for Hirschsprung disease, this patient is showing signs of an obstructive problem and all such patients require a contrast enema and an examination under anesthesia with rectal biopsy.

EUA

Intact dentate line and no stricture.

RECTAL BIOPSY

Normal; ganglion cells seen and no evidence of hypertrophies nerves (Remember: biopsy must be posterior in a Duhamel pull-through).

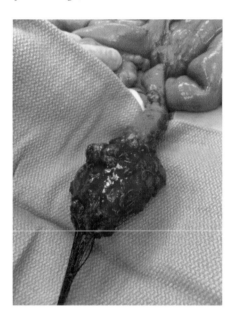

Figure 51.3 Clinical image. This child underwent a redo pull-through procedure involving resection of the Duhamel pouch. We felt the pouch itself was the cause of the obstruction. No spur was identified in the evaluation. The small bowel was also found to have been *twisted* at the time of the initial pull-through, as shown.

LEARNING POINT

- The complete workup of the child with obstructive symptoms following a pull-through procedure includes:
  - Repeat biopsy
  - Contrast enema
  - EUA
- The indications for a redo procedure in this child include:
  - Obstructive symptoms
  - Failure to thrive
  - Hirschsprung-associated enterocolitis episodes

ANSWER

51.1   B

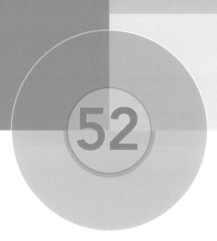

Seven-year-old boy with a history of Hirschsprung disease: Case study

52

CASE HISTORY

- A 7-year-old boy with a history of Hirschsprung disease (HD) who underwent a transanal Soave pull-through as an infant comes to see you because he has recurrent episodes of enterocolitis.
- At another institution, he underwent a redo of the pull-through because of a retained transition zone, but thereafter had no improvement of symptoms.
- A cecostomy was then performed to treat the continued obstructive symptoms, but without improvement. Finally, in desperation, an ileostomy was opened.
- The ileostomy was reversed, the obstructive symptoms returned, and it was reopened.
- You are asked to give an opinion.

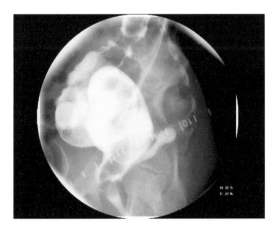

Figure 52.1 Contrast enema. What is your interpretation of the contrast enema?

REVIEW 52.1 MULTIPLE CHOICE QUESTION

What would be your advice with regards to the ongoing management of this child?

A. Colostomy

B. Ileostomy

C. Anorectal manometry

D. Examination under anesthesia of anus

Answer: This child has had a previous **Soave procedure** as demonstrated by the tract of contrast in the pelvis likely representing a cuff leak.

REVIEW 52.2 MULTIPLE CHOICE QUESTION

What do you find on examination?

A. Normal

B. Soave cuff

C. Damage to dentate line

D. Anastomotic stricture

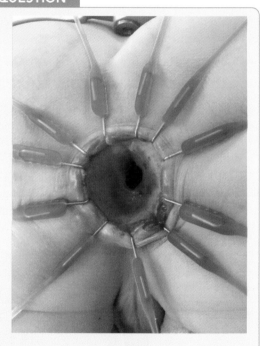

Figure 52.2 Transanal view showing extrinsic compression from Soave cuff.

MANAGEMENT

- This patient underwent a further redo procedure with resection of the Soave cuff.
- At 6-8 weeks, the ileostomy was closed after adequate healing of the redo pull-through and confirmation of no anastomotic stricture.
- Post-ileostomy closure, his chronic obstructive symptoms resolved. He is currently not on any medications and is not requiring cecostomy flushes. He has complete bowel control and the cecostomy was subsequently closed.

- Children with HD should be able to evacuate their bowels once the aganglionic bowel has been resected.
- If HD patients are having recurrent episodes of enterocolitis postoperatively, the immediate concern to the physician/surgeon should be that there is an anatomic or pathologic "problem" with the pull-through.
- This requires investigation as per the HD algorithm.

ANSWERS

52.1   D
52.2   B

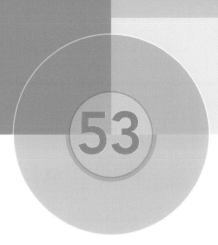

Twelve-year-old boy who underwent a Duhamel pull-through: Case study

53

CASE HISTORY

- A 12-year-old boy comes to your outpatient clinic for assessment. He has known Hirschsprung disease and underwent a Duhamel pull-through as a newborn with the transition zone being in the rectosigmoid.
- He developed multiple episodes of enterocolitis postoperatively, and this eventually resulted in him being managed with a defunctioning ileostomy at the age of 1 year.
- The original surgeons felt that the patient would benefit from a myotomy to relieve the obstructive symptoms and this was performed at 4 years of age. The ileostomy was reversed following the myotomy.

What are the risks of myotomy?

- After the ileostomy was reversed, he had continued fecal soiling, and therefore a cecostomy was performed at 10 years of age to allow for antegrade enemas. Bowel management with cecostomy flushes was not successful, and the patient continued to soil due to an inability to empty the colon.
- The Duhamel pouch was thought to be problematic, with failure to empty, and this was resected at 12 years of age and converted to a Swenson pull-through (coloanal anastomosis).
- He continues to have obstructive symptoms and recurrent episodes of enterocolitis.

MANAGEMENT

- **How are you going to manage this patient?**

MYOTOMY RISKS

- The risks of myotomy include fecal incontinence, fistula formation, and abscess.

MANAGEMENT

This patient requires full evaluation:

- Contrast enema
- Examination of anus under general anesthesia
- Repeat rectal biopsy to exclude a transition zone pull-through

REVIEW 53.1 MULTIPLE CHOICE QUESTION

What is your interpretation of this investigation?

A. Remnant of the Duhamel pouch
B. Normal
C. Hirschsprung-associated enterocolitis
D. Anastomotic stricture

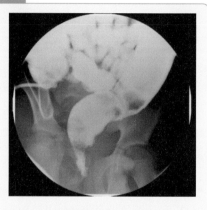

Figure 53.1 Contrast enema.

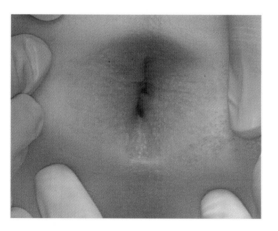

Figure 53.2 EUA findings. At examination, an extensive (1-cm thick circumferential) stricture was confirmed. Rectal biopsy was normal.

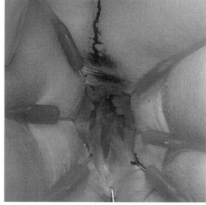

Figure 53.3 Intra-operative image. Extensive stricture.

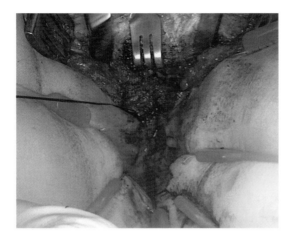

Figure 53.4 Stricture seen after placement of retraction pins and opening of posterior sagittal incision.

OPERATIVE NOTES

- The operative repair was via a posterior sagittal incision, which is sometimes required for a scarred rectum.
- The dentate line was preserved.
- An extensive stricture was resected, also requiring a laparotomy.
- A healthy segment of left colon was pulled through and anastomosed to the preserved anal canal (see Lane et al. 2016).
- A defunctioning ileostomy was performed to protect the anastomosis.
- The ileostomy was closed at 8 weeks postoperatively.
- The patient is well with no further episodes of enterocolitis and is clean.

REFERENCE

Lane VA et al. Rectal atresia and anal stenosis: The difference in the operative technique for these two distinct congenital anorectal malformations. *Tech Coloproctol* 2016; 20(4): 249–254.

ANSWER

53.1   D

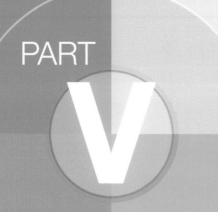

PART

V

FECAL INCONTINENCE AND CONSTIPATION

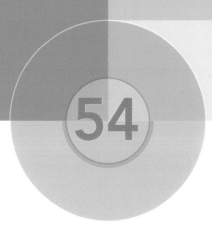

Introduction to bowel management

54

Fecal incontinence and constipation are major causes of morbidity in children with underlying colorectal problems including Hirschsprung disease and anorectal malformations. Functional (idiopathic) constipation with pseudo-incontinence (encopresis) is also a significant problem and is probably still underestimated, due to social embarrassment and lack of disclosure. Our algorithm for the care of this unique group is shown in Chapter 55. In addition, patients with spinal problems (e.g., spina bifida) can have problems with bowel control.

Bowel management is a term that is used to describe methods in which the bowel can be controlled in order to keep the patient clean or, expressed another way, socially continent.

There are various ways in which this can be achieved:

1. **Medical treatment:**
   a. For a slow-moving colon
      i. Laxatives
   b. For a fast-moving colon:
      i. Medication to slow colonic transit
      ii. Constipating diet and bulking agents (fiber)
2. **Mechanical treatment:**
   a. Enema program
      i. Rectal route
      ii. Antegrade enemas (via cecostomy or appendicostomy)

Each regimen must be tailored to the needs of the patient, with particular attention paid to the age of the child, the underlying diagnosis (e.g., Hirschsprung disease, anorectal malformation, functional constipation, spinal conditions, or sacrococcygeal teratoma) and the child's "potential" for bowel control (i.e., their inherent ability to have voluntary bowel movements).

A good potential for bowel control requires:

1. Maturity and commitment to potty training
2. Normal anatomy; anal canal and dentate line
3. Intact anal sphincters
4. Normal sacral anatomy
5. Normal spinal anatomy (and thus normal innervation of the anorectum)

6. An anoplasty (if a surgically created anus) located at the center of the sphincter mechanism *and* without stricture or prolapse

1. **Maturity and commitment to potty training:**
   a. The age of potty training varies from country to country. Certain areas will require the child be potty trained before the child can attend preschool or nursery school. There are therefore increasing social pressures for a child to be continent at a young age.
   b. Children with developmental delay from a variety of conditions such as Down's syndrome may not potty train on time, or ever, but they can still be socially clean with the appropriate bowel management regimen.
2. **Anal anatomy:**
   a. An intact anal canal is necessary anatomy for anal canal sensation and is required to recognize the difference between solid stool, liquid stool, and gas. In those with normal anatomy, these are recognized, controlled, and passed when socially acceptable, without leakage of stool.
   b. An additional factor is the inability to sense when the rectum is full (proprioception).
   c. This is likely based on feeling solid stool stretching the sphincter muscles.
   d. Anorectal malformation patients, in almost all cases, do not have a dentate line as their anal canal failed to develop and is therefore surgically created.
   e. The dentate line should be intact in Hirschsprung disease patients; however, it can be damaged during pull-through surgery if the dentate line is not preserved during the dissection.
   f. The dentate line may be damaged secondary to perineal trauma and in severe soft tissue infections.
3. **Anal sphincters:**
   a. The ability to squeeze the anus relies on the presence of intact anal sphincters, both voluntary (skeletal muscle) and involuntary (smooth muscle).
   b. The anal sphincters are normal in patients with idiopathic/functional constipation.
   c. In Hirschsprung disease, the quality of the sphincters is good, but they may not relax well. They are certainly not loose, unless overstretched and damaged during the pull-through procedure.
   d. The anal sphincters may be relatively normal in the patient with an anorectal malformation, with a good prognosis for bowel control, and these include the perineal fistulae, rectobulbar fistulae, vestibular fistulae, and short common channel cloaca patients.
   e. The anal sphincters may be more significantly affected (hypodeveloped) in the more severe anorectal malformations including rectoprostatic and bladder neck fistulae and long common channel and complex cloaca patients, rendering them less likely to achieve voluntary bowel control without bowel management therapies.
4. **Sacrum:**
   a. Hypodevelopment of the sacrum is commonly seen in patients with anorectal malformations and this can be objectively assessed by calculating a sacral ratio.
   b. The development of the sacrum seems to correlate with the development of the muscle and nerves of the pelvis. When foreshortened and hypodeveloped, so too are the sphincter muscles and nerves.
5. **Spinal cord:**
   a. Spinal defects can be seen in patients with anorectal malformations, spina bifida patients, those with a tethered spinal cord, occult spinal dysraphism, myelomeningocele, and in those with sacrococcygeal teratomas.

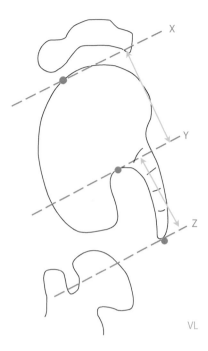

Figure 54.1 Sacral ratio measurement.

6. **Well-located anoplasty:**
    a. In patients with anorectal malformations, a key goal is to mobilize the distal rectum and to place the anoplasty/rectum in the center of the sphincter mechanism.
    b. In addition, ensuring that there is no rectal prolapse or rectal stricture is vital to maximizing the potential for bowel control.
    c. The anus needs to be in the correct anatomical location and without stricture or prolapse for the patient to be able to sense stool and for the sphincter mechanism to close adequately and relax at socially acceptable times.

WHY DO CHILDREN LEAK/SOIL/HAVE ACCIDENTS?

No child wants to be "dirty." The behavioral changes that occur when a child soils should be assumed to be as a result of the soiling, rather than vice versa. Children may require psychological support to deal with the negative effects that persistent soiling has had on their ability to form friendships and to cope with bullying. However, this is first and foremost a physiological problem that can secondarily become a psychological problem. The persistently soiling child can place enormous strain on a family and this can be in terms of extra financial burden, reduced social interactions, and difficulties in planning vacations due to soiling concerns, among many other examples.

BOWEL MANAGEMENT OPTIONS

Dietary modification to enhance constipation and bulk the stool:

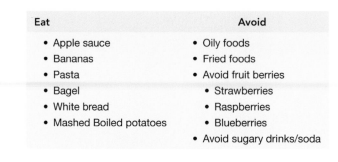

Eat	Avoid
• Apple sauce	• Oily foods
• Bananas	• Fried foods
• Pasta	• Avoid fruit berries
• Bagel	• Strawberries
• White bread	• Raspberries
• Mashed Boiled potatoes	• Blueberries
	• Avoid sugary drinks/soda

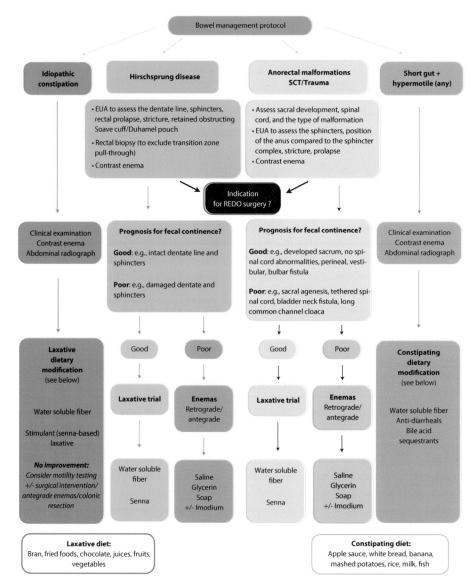

Figure 54.2 Bowel management algorithm.

Adjusting the diet can be very useful in certain patient groups, particularly ileoanal pull-through patients. A constipating diet can provide bulk and help to reduce the frequency of the stool.

FIBER: SOLUBLE AND INSOLUBLE

- Soluble fiber (e.g., pectin) binds water and forms bulkier stool. This can be beneficial in the anorectal malformation group of patients in particular, as it helps with the sensation of stool.
- Insoluble fiber (e.g., methylcellulose) does not absorb water, but has the capacity to bind with bile acid. This form of fiber tends to make the stool soft. This can actually reduce the patient's capacity to feel the stool if it is too soft/loose.

STOOL SOFTENERS (POLYETHYLENE GLYCOL/DIOCTYL SODIUM SULFOSUCCINATE)

- As the name suggests, these medications soften the stool. Polyethylene glycol is an osmotic laxative, drawing water into the bowel lumen.
- Dioctyl sodium sulfosuccinate is an anionic detergent that has been shown to stimulate water and electrolyte secretion.
- Soft/mushy stool can be difficult to feel and empty. In anorectal malformation patients, stool softeners should not be used.

STIMULANT LAXATIVES (SENNA/BISACODYL)

- The breakdown products of senna cause irritation of the colonic wall, leading it to induce fluid secretion and colonic contraction.
- Bisacodyl has two mechanisms of action:
  - It is a contact laxative and increases fluid and NaCl secretion.
  - It stimulates the enteric nerves to cause colonic mass movements (this is one of the reasons it is used in colonic manometry as it stimulates the colon to contract).

ANTI-DIARRHEALS (LOPERAMIDE HYDROCHLORIDE)

- Loperamide is an opioid receptor agonist and acts on the μ-opioid receptors in the myenteric plexus of the intestine, but does not affect the central nervous system. The mechanism of action is to reduce the activity of the myenteric plexus, which in turn decreases the tone of the circular and longitudinal smooth muscles of the intestinal wall, thus increasing the time that the digested material remains in the large intestine, allowing for more water to be reabsorbed. Loperamide also suppresses gastrocolic reflex, thereby decreasing colonic mass movements.
- Diphenoxylate and atropine combinations (e.g., Lomotil). Diphenoxylate is an opioid agonist and acts as an anti-diarrheal agent by slowing intestinal contractions and peristalsis (atropine is added to prevent overdose as this causes tachycardia).

ELECTROLYTE IMBALANCE (ZINC DEFICIENCY)

- Malnutrition is recognized to be a major factor in the etiology, management, and prognosis of persistent diarrhea in young children. The risk of zinc deficiency is increased in children with diarrhea, and it is recognized that mild to severe zinc deficiency can contribute to the severity and duration of diarrheal disease, resulting in a vicious cycle. Adding zinc if a patient is deficient can improve the diarrhea.

CHOLESTYRAMINE/COLESTIPOL (BILE ACID SEQUESTRANT)

Chronic diarrhea may be caused by excess bile acids entering the colon, rather than being absorbed in the ileum. This can be a primary idiopathic condition or secondary to surgical resection or inflammatory bowel disease. Bile acid sequestrants bind the excess bile acids, thereby reducing diarrhea. Care must be taken in their use due to significant drug interactions and also the binding of fat-soluble vitamins, which could lead to vitamin A, D, and E deficiency.

ENEMA CONSTITUENTS

GLYCEROL/GLYCERINE POLYOL (SUGAR ALCOHOL) COMPOUND

- When inserted into the colon via an enema, the glycerol irritates the colonic mucosa and induces a hyperosmolar effect.

SOAPSUDS (E.G., CASTILE SOAP; A VEGETABLE OIL-BASED SOAP)

- Soap suds can increase the effectiveness of the enema. There are rare case reports in the literature describing patients who have developed a detergent colitis/proctitis following soap enema use, but in the majority this approach is well tolerated.

FURTHER READING

Harish K et al. Severe colitis induced by soap enemas. *Indian J Gastroenterol* 2006; 25(2): 99–100.

Moriarty KJ et al. Studies on the mechanism of action of dioctyl sodium sulphosuccinate in the human jejunum. *Gut* 1985; 26: 1008–1013.

Orchard JL, Lawson R. Severe colitis induced by soap enemas. *South Med J* 1986; 79(11): 1459–1460.

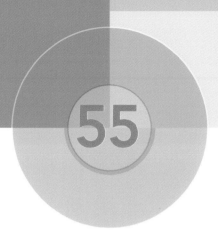

Idiopathic/functional constipation: Management algorithm

55

- **Maximal medical therapy failed:**
- Continued constipation
- Persistent soiling/accidents
- Abdominal pain
- Intolerance of medication due to side effects

- Failure to thrive
- Young patient <3 yrs
- Diffuse colonic dysmotility on colonic manometry

- Ileostomy

- Repeat colonic manometry in 1–2 years

- IAS Achalsia
- EAS dyssynergia
- Severe withholding

- **Botox**
  - Internal anal sphincter (IAS)
  - External anal sphincter (EAS)
  - Or both IAS and EAS

- Constipation with fecal impaction
- **No soiling**

- Laparoscopic resection based on **colonic manometry** findings (usually sigmoid +/- left colon)

- Constipation with fecal impaction
- **Soiling**

- Laparoscopic resection based on colonic manometry findings (usually sigmoid and left colon) + Malone appendicostomy/cecostomy
- **Aim**: to reduce time of flushes and reduce future laxative requirements

---

- Success with rectal enemas but child unable to tolerate per rectal administration

- Colonic manometry normal
- Cecostomy only and **retest after one year** with laxative trial

---

- Failure with cecostomy/rectal enemas.
- Failure following colonic resection and antegrade flushes.

- Repeat colonic manometry and consider further colonic resection based on findings.

- Consider sacral nerve stimulator

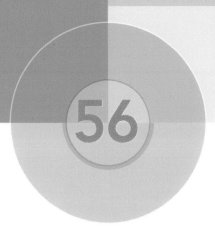

CASE HISTORY

- A 4-year-old girl presents to your outpatient clinic.
- She was born with an anorectal malformation (rectovestibular fistula) that was repaired when she was 3 months old.
- As part of her VACTERL screening she was found to have:
  - Tethered cord: Released at the age of 1 year
  - Hemisacrum
  - Solitary left kidney with lower pole scarring
- She presents with constipation and fecal incontinence.

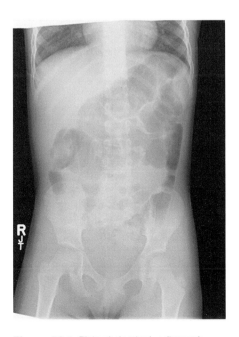

Figure 56.1 Plain abdominal radiograph.

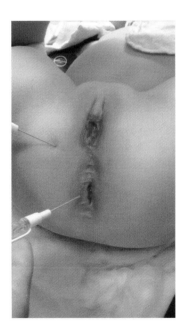

Figure 56.2 Examination of perineum.

Where is the anus positioned?

A. Within the sphincter complex

B. Partially in the sphincter complex

C. Outside the sphincter complex

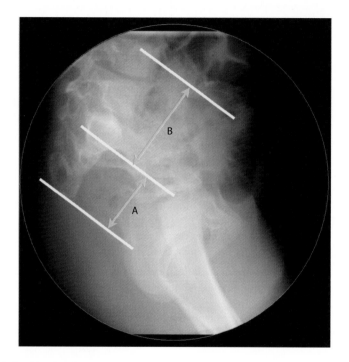

Figure 56.3 Lateral image of sacrum.

What does the contrast enema show?

A. Normal

B. Stricture

C. Pre-sacral mass

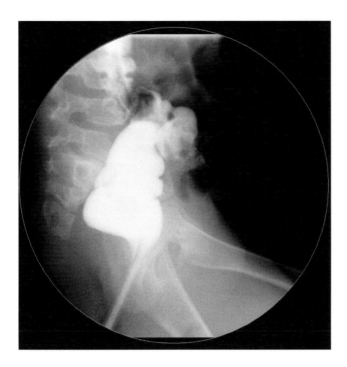

Figure 56.4 Lateral image of contrast study.

REVIEW 56.3 MULTIPLE CHOICE QUESTION

What is the sacral ratio in Figure 56.3. A = 2.6 cm, B = 6 cm?

A. 0.37
B. 2.14
C. 0.43
D. 0.96

REVIEW 56.4 MULTIPLE CHOICE QUESTION

What is the likely potential for fecal continence in this patient at present, given the anatomy and the radiological information?

A. Excellent potential
B. Good potential
C. Poor potential

LEARNING POINTS

- This child has a poor potential for bowel control.
  - She has a history of tethered cord and a sacral ratio that is in the intermediate range.
  - The anus is mislocated.
  - Her potential for bowel control is likely to improve with a redo primary posterior sagittal anorectoplasty (PSARP) and correction of the anatomy.
- We decided to manage her prior to her redo surgery with rectal enemas, but at the age of 4 years, she did not tolerate these well at home.
- She then underwent the redo PSARP and is currently clean with one stool a day on stimulant laxatives and water-soluble fiber.

ANSWERS

56.1   C
56.2   A
56.3   C
56.4   B

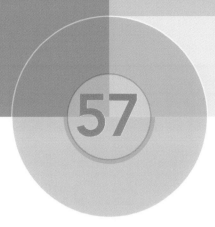

Anorectal malformation and soiling: Case study

57

CASE HISTORY

- A 5-year-old boy is assessed for fecal incontinence.
- He was born with an anorectal malformation and a rectourethral fistula (level unknown).
- He was managed initially with a colostomy, then underwent a primary posterior sagittal anorectoplasty (PSARP) at 1 year of age, and the colostomy has since been reversed.
- The mother reports that she has tried rectal enemas previously without success, and the child's current regimen is 45 mg of senna.
- He has abdominal cramping and vomiting after taking the senna and continues to have accidents throughout the day.
- He is incontinent of urine (day and night). No attempts have been made to potty train.

INVESTIGATIONS

- On **physical examination** in the outpatient department, the anus was noted to be:
  - Small (calibrated to a size 8 Hegar)
  - Posteriorly mislocated
  - Prolapsed (minor)
- **Renal ultrasound**: Normal.
- **Sacral radiograph**: Normal. Sacral ratio 0.71.
- **Magnetic resonance imaging of the spine**: No spinal cord tethering.
- **Magnetic resonance imaging of the pelvis**: Normal. No evidence of a remnant of the original fistula (ROOF).
- **Contrast study**: Non-dilated colon.
- Bowel management program is begun.

REVIEW 57.1 MULTIPLE CHOICE QUESTION

What is your assessment of his continence potential?

A. Poor
B. Good

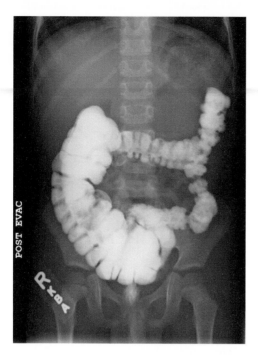

Figure 57.1 Day 1: Contrast enema, non-dilated colon. Based on this Contrast study we judge the first day's enema to be: Initial regimen: 400 mL saline and 20 mL glycerin.

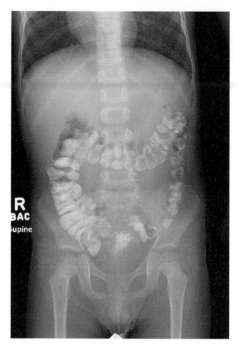

Figure 57.2 Day 2: Small amount of residual contrast colon cleared of stool by yesterday's enema. Parents report that child passed one stool and had an episode of smearing. Plan: Regimen increased to 400 mL saline and 25 mL glycerin.

LEARNING POINTS

- This child has a good potential for bowel control. His sacral ratio is 0.71 and he has a normal spine.
- His self-confidence will be much improved by being clean on enemas for several months.
- The patient returned for a redo PSARP to improve the anatomy and the potential for continence. He also has a Malone appendicostomy fashioned to allow antegrade administration of the same enema regimen and, when more mature, he may succeed with a laxative trial, and could ultimately not need a mechanical system to empty the colon.

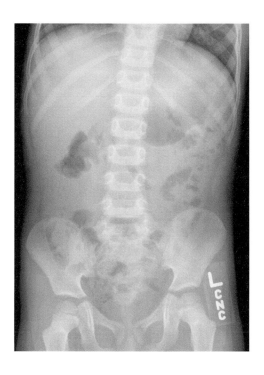

Figure 57.3 Parents report an accident 1 hour after the enema had been administered. Abdominal radiograph demonstrates moderate stool in the descending colon and rectum. Regimen: 400 mL saline/30 mL glycerin.

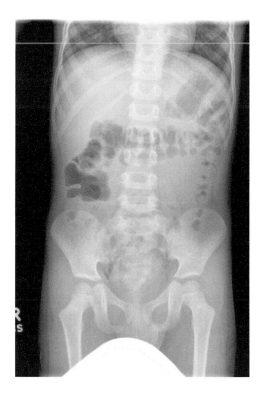

Figure 57.4 Day 3: Parents report no accidents and no abdominal cramping. Abdominal radiograph demonstrates no stool in the descending colon or rectum. Regimen: continued the same.

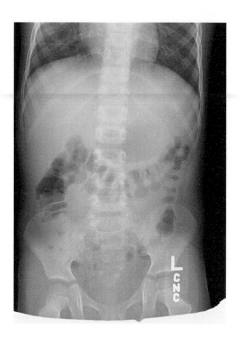

Figure 57.5 Day 4: Parents report one bowel movement after the enema, no accidents, and no abdominal cramping. Radiograph shows some stool in the rectum. Regimen: 400 mL saline and 30 mL glycerin.

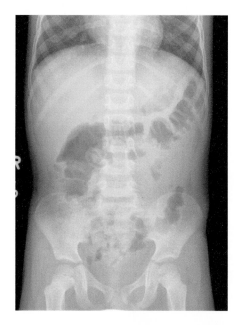

Figure 57.6 Abdominal radiograph demonstrates no stool in the colon or rectum. Final regimen: 400 mL saline and 30 mL glycerin.

ANSWER

57.1   B

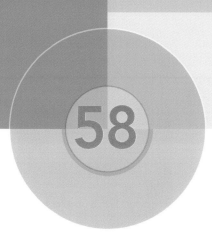

Bowel management—Appendicostomy flush: Case study

58

CASE HISTORY

- This is a case of a teenage boy with an anorectal malformation.
- He underwent a posterior sagittal anorectoplasty (PSARP) for an anorectal malformation with no fistula as a baby following an initial colostomy, and then a colostomy closure.
- He required a redo PSARP (for a rectal stricture) with covering colostomy at the age of 6 years.
- The colostomy was reversed 8 weeks postoperatively and a cecostomy was placed.
- He recovered well from these operations and was under routine follow-up. His cecostomy was converted to a Malone appendicostomy electively.
- He performs intermittent urethral catheterization for a neurogenic bladder.
- He presents to clinic for follow-up and reports that he is having increasing problems with the Malone appendicostomy.
- Flushes taking ≥2 hours to complete and are associated with abdominal pain and cramping. He has intermittent soiling as well.

REVIEW 58.1 MULTIPLE CHOICE QUESTION

How are you going to investigate this child?

A. Contrast study, via the Malone
B. Sitz marker study

REVIEW 58.2 MULTIPLE CHOICE QUESTION

What is this child's potential for fecal continence?

A. Very good

B. 50:50

C. Very poor

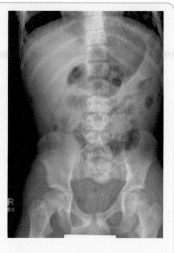

Figure 58.1 Plan x-ray.

You note a poor sacrum consistent with poor potential for bowel control.

REVIEW 58.3 MULTIPLE CHOICE QUESTION

What is considered an acceptable/normal length of time required for a cecostomy/appendicostomy flush?

A. Immediate response

B. 15 minutes

C. 45–60 minutes

D. 60–90 minutes

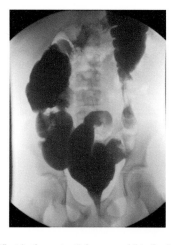

Figure 58.2 Contrast enema. What is the potential cause of this finding on the contrast enema? There is a stricture, probably at the site of the previous colostomy, closure site, which requires resection.

- A Malone flush should take **45–60 minutes** to complete.
- If it is taking longer than this, the child needs further assessment. Contrast via the Malone simulates the flush and provides a lot of information.

1. Is there a colonic stricture?
2. Is there a rectal stricture?
3. Do the flush constituents need to be altered?
4. Is there redundancy of the colon requiring resection?

ANSWERS

58.1	A
58.2	C
58.3	C

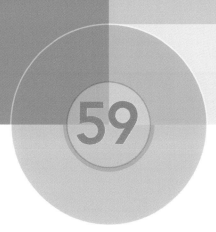

Bowel management— Antegrade flush: Case study

59

- You are asked to see a 5-year-old boy who was born with an anorectal malformation and spina bifida occulta.
- The anorectal malformation (perineal fistula) was repaired in the newborn period.
- He developed severe constipation at the age of 2 years, which did not respond to high doses of laxatives.
- At the age of 4 years he had a cecostomy placed.
- At the time of review in your clinic he was receiving the following cecostomy flush:
  - 1400 mL saline
  - 30 mL glycerin
  - 40 mL soap
  - Stool softeners
- He was not clean with the above regimen and the flushes were taking 1.5 hours.
- Often he would retain the flush until the next day and have frequent daytime soiling accidents.

What other information would you like to know?

What are the factors that determine his potential for continence?

- Spina bifida occulta (no tethered cord)
- Sacral ratio 0.65
- Original malformation was a perineal fistula

You perform an examination of the perineum and find:

- A well-located anus within the muscle complex
- No prolapse or stricture
- Good musculature

POTENTIAL FOR FECAL CONTINENCE AND PLAN

- This patient has a good potential for bowel control, even with his past medical history of spina bifida occulta.

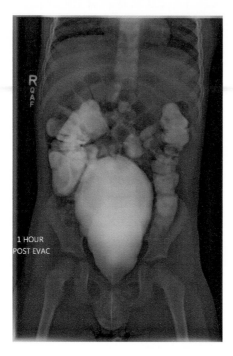

Figure 59.1 Contrast via the cecostomy. What is your interpretation of the contrast study?

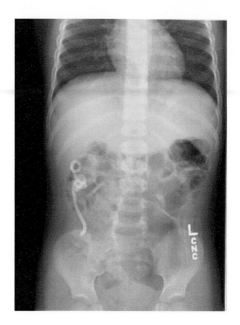

Figure 59.2 Bowel management radiographs. Day 1: dilated rectosigmoid persists following contrast study. Large doses of senna introduced with limited success. Cecostomy flush still required.

- His original anorectal malformation carries a good prognosis for bowel control and he has had a good anatomical repair, normal spine, and a "medium" sacral ratio.
- His dilated rectosigmoid likely relates to inadequate management of his constipation when he was a toddler.
- He was entered into the bowel management program and the cecostomy flush was adjusted. He then continued to a laxative trial.

REVIEW 59.1 MULTIPLE CHOICE QUESTION

How would you manage this patient? The cecostomy flushes are failing to empty the rectum and the patient has failed a laxative trial.

A. Left-sided colon (distal) antegrade continence enema (ACE)

B. Resect pouch and perform a coloanal anastomosis

C. Resect the pouch, leaving the distal rectum, and perform a colorectal anastomosis

D. Colostomy

FURTHER READING

Eradi B et al. The role of colonic resection in combination with a Malone appendicostomy as part of the bowel management program for the treatment of fecal incontinence. *J Ped Surg* 2013; 48: 2296–2300.

ANSWER

59.1   C

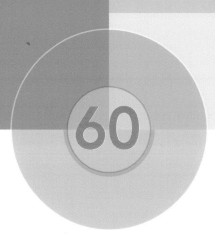

Patient with functional constipation and failed medical management: Case study

CASE HISTORY

- This is the case of a 15-year-old girl with functional constipation.
- She developed problems with constipation at a young age, and this has been managed with high-dose stimulant laxatives and enemas, resulting in bowel movements only twice weekly, and she suffers from daytime soiling.
- The patient is failing to tolerate the stimulant laxatives (150–200 mg of senna daily) and is experiencing severe abdominal cramps on a daily basis.

MANAGEMENT PLAN

- She had previously failed medical therapy, but we reconfirmed this with an intensive bowel management program for 1 week.

What else would you like to know, and are there any investigations that you would like to perform?

Contrast enema

Slightly redundant colon

Mildly dilated rectum

- She repeated the laxative trial with water-soluble fiber without success. She continued to have intolerance to laxatives.
- We therefore suspected that she may have had abnormal colonic motility and we performed colonic manometry.

COLONIC MANOMETRY

- Fasting phase: Multiple phasic and tonic contractions with hyperactive colon.
- Post-prandial phase: The colon continued to have uncoordinated contractions, with no evidence of propagating contractions.
- Stimulant challenge: Abdominal cramping was experienced, but there was no evidence of high-amplitude propagating contractions in keeping with an inert colon.

MANAGEMENT PLAN

After discussion with the parent and family, we elected to perform a laparoscopic colonic resection of the proximal rectum and sigmoid with the majority of the rectum being spared (the rectum is required to maximize the continence potential, with a Malone appendicostomy for antegrade flushes. She can then undergo a repeat laxative trial in the future (Gasior et al., 2016).

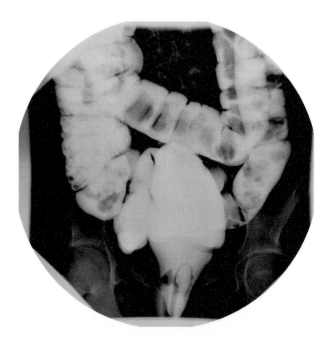

Figure 60.1 Contrast enema. Non-dilated but redundant colon demonstrated.

LEARNING POINTS

- It is important to look at the contrast enema for colonic dilation, but also to appreciate possible colonic redundancy if the patient is resistant to high-dose laxatives or experiences severe side effects.
- Colonic manometry is a useful guide to determine resection once one concludes that the patient has failed medical management. Collaboration with the GI motility team is key to helping these patients.

REFERENCE

Gasior A, Brisighelli G, Diefenbach K, Lane VA, Reck C, Wood RJ, Levitt MA. Surgical management of functional constipation: Preliminary report of a new approach using a laparoscopic sigmoid resection combined with a Malone appendicostomy. *Eur J Pediatr Surg* 2016; Oct 25. [Epub ahead of print].

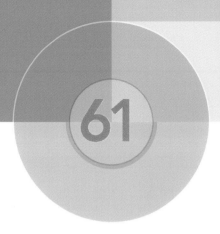

Bowel management for fecal incontinence: Case study

61

- A 12-year-old female with rectovestibular fistula is receiving daily antegrade enemas via a cecostomy.
- She has a past medical history of
  - VATER syndrome
  - Vesicoureteral reflux
  - Hemivaginas with vaginal septum (removed during the PSARP)
- She initially presented to your outpatient clinic on a flush regimen of
  - 500 mL normal saline
  - 10 mg bisacodyl
- The whole process was taking 3–4 hours before feeling empty, but she continued to have fecal accidents throughout the day.
- Her contrast enema shows dilatation of the right colon but is otherwise normal.

The first thing that needs to be clarified is whether the anatomy is normal. She was old enough to be examined in the office. There was a normally sited anus within the sphincters and no stricture.

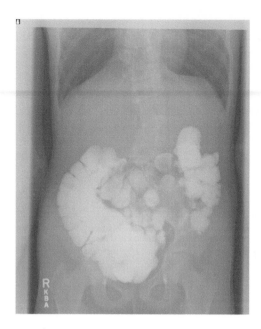

Figure 61.1 Contrast enema.

REVIEW 61.1 MULTIPLE CHOICE QUESTION

How would you manage this child's bowel management?

A. Laxatives
B. Change the antegrade flush regimen
C. Rectal enemas

LEARNING POINTS

- This child was initially managed with a change in her antegrade flush regimen to:
  - 500 mL normal saline
  - 20 mg glycerin
- This regimen was successful and the flush time reduced to 45–60 minutes.
- The bisacodyl was likely provoking accidents given its stimulant activity.
- She was clean with this regimen, which increased her confidence, and she returned for a laxative trial.

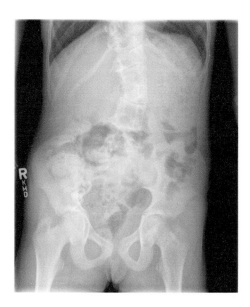

Figure 61.2 Bowel management radiographs. Day 1: laxative trial commenced: on three squares (45 mg) of senna and two tablespoons of water-soluble fiber.

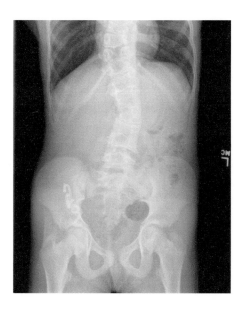

Figure 61.3 Abdominal x-ray. Day 2: Mom reports she had four total bowel movements in the morning with no accidents or soiling, but only took one tablespoon of fiber. Decreased to 2.5 squares of senna (37.5 mg) and encouraged to take two tablespoons of water-soluble fiber to help bulk up the stool to aim for one to two stools daily. A laxative diet was also encouraged.

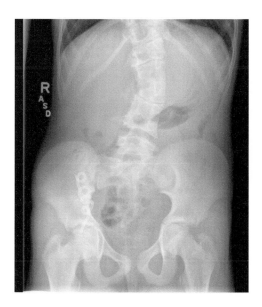

Figure 61.4 X-ray day 1. Mom reports she had four bowel movements during the day with no accidents or soiling. Recommendation to increase the fiber to three tablespoons and continue with 2.5 squares of senna and a laxative diet. She remained clean with one to two well-formed stools on the last 2 days in the program. Final regimen: three tablespoons of water-soluble fiber, 2.5 squares of senna, and a laxative diet.

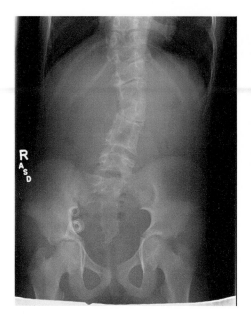

Figure 61.5 X-ray showing a clean colon. Day 6: Clean colon.

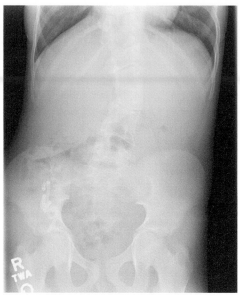

Figure 61.6 X-ray showing a clean colon, successful regimen. Day 7: Clean colon, successful regimen.

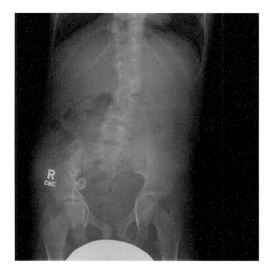

Figure 61.7 X-ray showing a clean colon. 1 month: Clean colon.

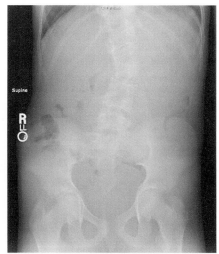

Figure 61.8 X-ray showing a clean colon. 3 months: She remains successful on two squares of Senna, two tablespoons of water-soluble fiber, and a laxative diet. Her cecostomy has been removed.

ANSWER

61.1   B

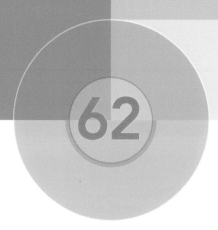
Rectovestibular fistula and soiling: Case study

CASE HISTORY

- A 5-year-old female attends the clinic for bowel management.
- She was born with a rectovestibular fistula that was surgically corrected at birth in another institution.
- She is fecally incontinent and has reduced potential for bowel control due to sacral agenesis (sacral ratio <0.4).
- In discussion with the parents, and given the age of the patient, a rectal enema regimen was decided on in the first instance to "get the patient clean," with the eventual aim of a laxative trial when she is older.

ASSESSMENT OF PREVIOUS REPAIR

INVESTIGATIONS

- Examination under anesthesia of the anus:
  - Normal position of the anus within the sphincter complex
  - No evidence of prolapse
  - No stricture
- Cystovaginoscopy:
  - Normal bladder with no evidence of trabeculation
  - Normal vaginal introitus
  - Cervix seen with mucous
- Contrast enema:
  - Assess anatomy of the colon
  - See Figure 62.1

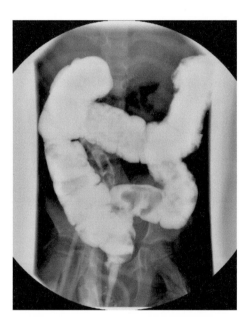

Figure 62.1 Contrast enema. Normal appearance of the colon from the rectum to the cecum. Day 1: Parents had difficulty with the first rectal enema. A Foley catheter was used to instill the enema and the balloon was deflated too soon, and the solution leaked with very little stool. Parents were re-educated.

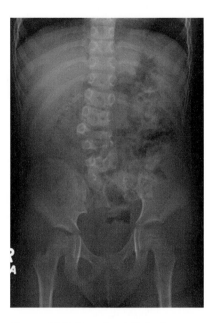

Figure 62.2 X-ray day 1. Patient reported abdominal cramps with administration of the rectal enema. Parents instructed to slow the rate of instillation of the enema solution. No accidents reported today. Radiograph shows stool throughout the colon. No changes made to rectal enema constituents today.

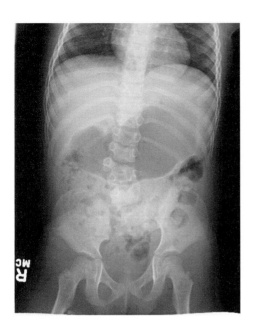

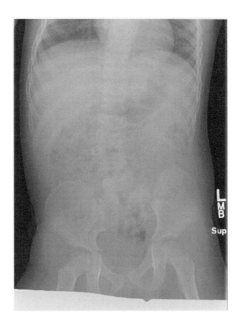

Figure 62.3 Abdominal x-ray. Days 3 and 4: Parents report that the patient has been clean with no accidents. No changes made to the regimen.

Figure 62.4 Abdominal x-ray. Day 5: Parents report a small accident overnight. The regimen was altered. New regimen: saline 400 mL, glycerin reduced to 5 mL, (to make the enema a little weaker) and two tablespoon of water-soluble fiber added to diet.

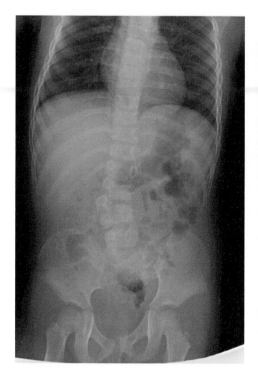

Figure 62.5 Abdominal x-ray. Day 6: No accidents, therefore continuation of the current regimen.

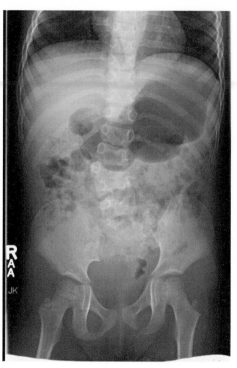

Figure 62.6 Abdominal x-ray. Day 7: Small accident overnight. Increased fecal loading on the radiograph. Regimen changed: saline 450 mL, glycerin 20 mL, and stopped the fiber, as it may have been causing too much bulk.

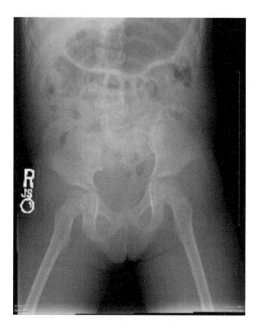

Figure 62.7 Abdominal x-ray. Day 30: Patient continues on the same regimen with no concerns or complaints from parents and no accidents. Final regimen: saline 450 mL and glycerin 20 mL. Patient remains clean.

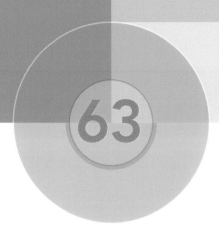

Bowel management program for soiling: Case study

63

CASE HISTORY

- A 12-year-old girl with anorectal malformation and a rectovestibular fistula, which was repaired in the newborn period, attends your clinic for further management.
- She has the following **associated malformations**:
  - Esophageal atresia
  - Vesicoureteric reflux
  - Spinal hemivertebrae and scoliosis
- There is no evidence of a sacral anomaly (sacral ratio 0.75) and no tethered cord was found on spinal imaging in the newborn period.
- When she was 8 years old (4 years ago) she was having fecal incontinence and daily soiling.
- A cecostomy was performed and antegrade enemas initiated.
- The cecostomy flushes are reported to take 3–4 hours to complete and she continues to have problems with daily soiling.

How would you proceed with the management of this patient?

What else needs to be considered given the history?

TO BE CONSIDERED

1. What is the anatomy like?
2. What is her chance of achieving continence?
3. Why are the flushes taking 3–4 hours? What flush constituents is she currently using?
4. Is she fecally impacted and suffering from overflow incontinence?

- She had examination under anesthesia of the anus and this demonstrated an excellent result from previous rectovestibular repair.
- The anus was sited within the sphincter complex and there was no evidence of a stricture and therefore nothing to suggest a distal bowel obstruction, and no rectal prolapse.
- This patient should have an excellent chance of achieving bowel control. Her original malformation was a rectovestibular fistula with no associated sacral/spinal abnormalities.

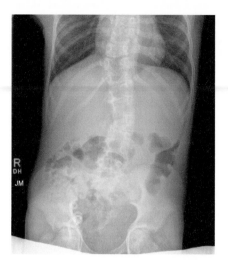

Figure 63.1 Plain radiograph.

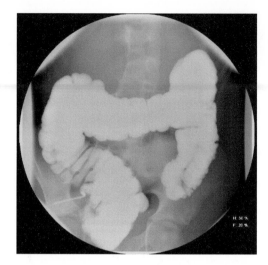

Figure 63.2 Contrast study via the cecostomy.

- The flush simply contained saline, with no added medications.
- Her abdominal radiograph is shown in Figure 63.1. The cecostomy is evident and there is moderate fecal loading apparent.
- You decide to perform a contrast enema (via the cecostomy), which is shown in Figure 63.2 to watch the flow of the cecostomy flush.
- The contrast study via the cecostomy does not show any significant hold up to explain why the flush regimen is taking 3-4 hours, which is important to establish.
- With this knowledge, it is appropriate to adjust the flush constituents to make it more effective.

PLAN

- The cecostomy flush was changed to make it more "powerful"—450 mL saline and 20 mL glycerin—with excellent results.
- The time for the flush was reduced to 45 minutes with the addition of glycerin and she was clean within 48 hours, with no soiling.
- Once she was clean and confident, given her excellent potential for bowel control and good anorectal repair, she returned for a bowel management program with a trial of laxatives.

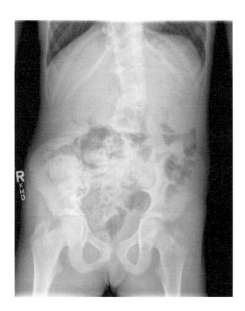

Figure 63.3 Bowel management program—days 1, 3, and 6. No fecal loading in the descending colon, and therefore commenced laxative trial of senna and water-soluble fiber.

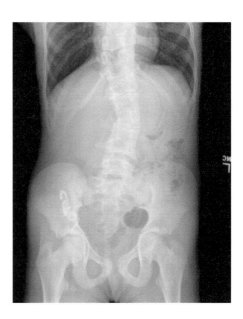

Figure 63.4 Abdominal x-ray. Day 3: Patient had been commenced on two squares of senna (chocolate square preparation equal to 30 mg of senna) and two tablespoons of water-soluble fiber which provides bulks and avoids the laxatives from causing watery stools.

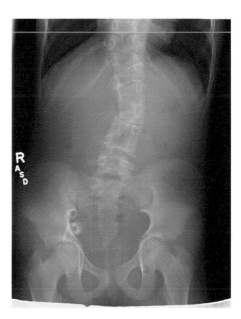

Figure 63.5 Abdominal x-ray. Day 6: Empty colon on same regimen. Clean x-ray and clean patient. Successful laxative regimen.

LEARNING POINTS

1. Be sure to review the history carefully in any patient that presents to your clinic and assess for potential for bowel control.
2. The postoperative anatomy of any child with a previous anorectal malformation repair needs to be checked for position of the anus and for evidence of a stricture or a rectal prolapse, all of which may warrant repair to provide the best possible anatomy to reach their continence potential.
3. If the cecostomy flush is taking an excessive amount of time, the anatomy of the colon must be established. For example, there may be a colonic stricture from a previous colostomy takedown/reversal that is causing delayed transit. In this case, the flush was simply not strong enough (stimulating enough) to clean the colon.
4. Ultimately, this patient did not need a cecostomy at all, as she had excellent potential for bowel control and was able to be clean on laxatives alone, capable of her own voluntary bowel movements. After successful laxative trial her cecostomy was closed.

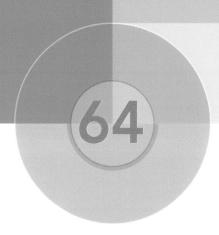

Rectal prolapse: Case study

CASE HISTORY

- A 3-year-old boy presents to your clinic with a 7-week history of recurrent rectal prolapse.
- He has a history of constipation and has been on a stool softener and stimulant laxative, with no improvements in his symptoms.
- There is no past surgical history.
- The prolapse is causing discomfort, and the child is becoming reluctant to eat.

What else would you like to know, and are there any investigations you would consider?

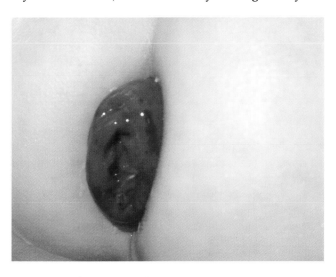

Figure 64.1 Clinical image. Rectal prolapse.

TO CONSIDER

1. Is there a chronic history of constipation and straining?
2. Has there been a recent gastroenteritis episode?

3. What is the child's diet? Is the child malnourished?
4. Is there a history of cystic fibrosis?
5. Has there been recent travel? Parasitic infection?
6. Is there a pelvic/pre-sacral mass?
7. Is there any history to suggest inflammatory bowel disease?
8. Is there a history of a connective tissue disorder?
9. Are there any spinal problems?

INVESTIGATIONS TO CONSIDER

1. Nutritional assessment
2. Abdominal radiograph to assess constipation ± contrast enema
3. Sweat test for cystic fibrosis (El-Chammas et al. 2015)
4. Stool for culture and parasites
5. Magnetic resonance imaging of the spine to rule out any spinal anomaly or any presacral mass
6. Colonoscopy to assess for inflammatory bowel disease and biopsies
7. Genetic screening if clinically indicated

Surgical options: There are many surgical options for the management of rectal prolapse. The surgeon's choice of operation will depend on the patient's age, the underlying cause of the prolapse, and the surgeon's experience. Options include

1. Theirsch suture
2. Injection of sclerosing agents (mucosal prolapse)
3. Altemeier procedure
4. Delorme procedure
5. Transanal rectal resection
6. Rectopexy

LEARNING POINTS

1. Rectal prolapse is common and often resolves with adequate medical treatment of constipation and dietary modification.
2. The physician, however, needs to be aware of conditions predisposing to prolapse of the rectum, including cystic fibrosis.
3. Underlying causes of severe constipation must be treated as a first step.
4. Other causes including a pre-sacral mass, spinal lesion, or pelvic mass must also be ruled out.
5. Our preference once all other factors have been ruled out and constipation adequately treated is to perform a transanal Swenson rectal resection of 6 to 8 cm of rectum.

SUGGESTED READING

El-Chammas KI et al. Rectal prolapse and cystic fibrosis. *J Pediatr Gastroenterol Nutr* 2015; 60: 110–112.

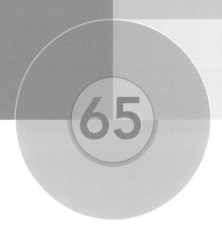

65

Functional constipation: Case study

CASE HISTORY

- A 6-year-old male with a long-standing history of functional (idiopathic) constipation is referred to you by the gastroenterologist who believes he needs surgical intervention.
- The patient has tried multiple medical regimens without success, including:
  - Miralax (stool softener) 1 capful
  - Bisacodyl 5 mg in the morning
  - Fleet enemas as needed
- The mother reports that the child has an awareness of needing to stool, but occasionally gets "backed up" and does experience smearing several times a week.
- He passes formed stools two to three times per week.

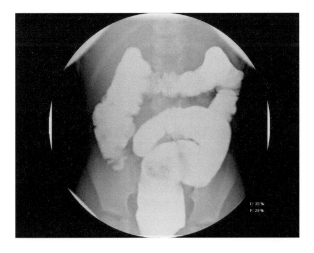

Figure 65.1 Contrast enema. Normal colonic anatomy (other than a redundant sigmoid) and moderate stool descending the rectum.

How would you manage this child's constipation?

A. Rectal enemas

B. Laxative (stimulant) regimen

C. Stool softeners

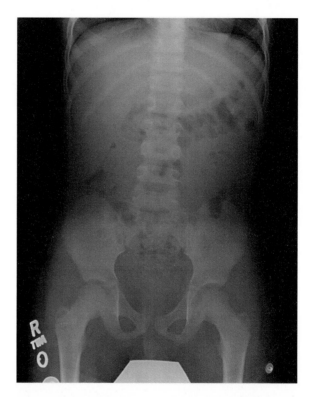

Figure 65.2 Bowel management radiographs. Day 1: Stool demonstrated in the rectum. Therefore, the patient was given a Fleet enema to empty the colon, and then the patient was commenced on chocolate senna (3.5 squares/52.5 mg) and two tablespoons of water-soluble fiber which provides bulk and avoids the watery nature of stool the laxative can provoke. This patient is suitable for a stimulant laxative trial. He has functional constipation and therefore good potential for bowel control, is at an age where he has good understanding, and should be motivated to be clean and in normal underwear.

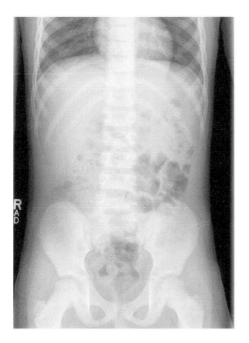

Figure 65.3 Abdominal x-ray: Clean colon.

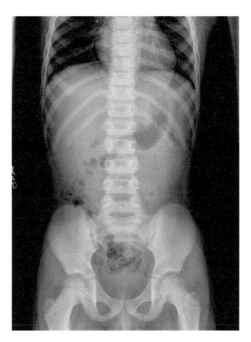

Figure 65.4 Abdominal x-ray: Some stool in rectum.

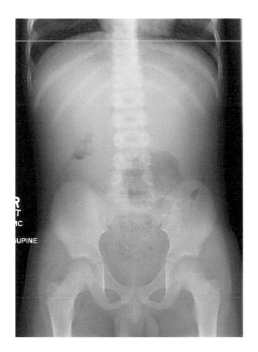

Figure 65.5 Abdominal x-ray: Clean colon, except stool in rectum.

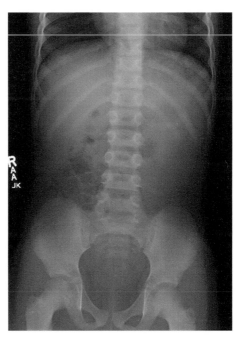

Figure 65.6 Abdominal x-ray: Clean colon, final image—clean patient.

ANSWER

65.1   B

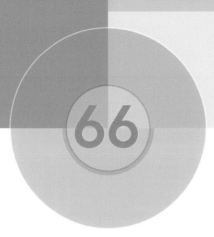

Bowel management for a patient with spina bifida: Case study

66

- An 11-year-old female with a past medical history of spina bifida.
- She is continent of urine, and voids spontaneously. These facts are encouraging for her potential to also have fecal continence.
- She developed significant constipation at the age of 9 years and was found to have tethering of the spinal cord, which has been released.
- She attends the bowel management program for constipation and soiling.

How would you manage this child?

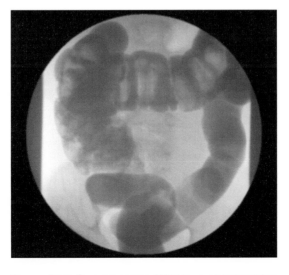

Figure 66.1 Contrast enema. What is your interpretation of this contrast study?

The colon is non-dilated and there is no evidence of a redundant rectosigmoid. The non-dilatation is likely due to poor innervation. The colon can still be hypomotile.

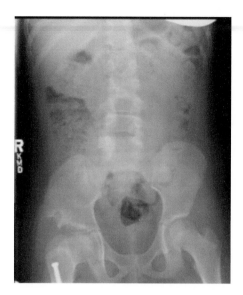

Figure 66.2 Bowel management radiographs. Day 1: We decided to manage this patient with rectal enemas. What would your starting rectal enema be (i.e., volume and constituents)?

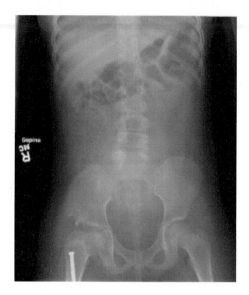

Figure 66.3 Abdominal x-ray Day 2.

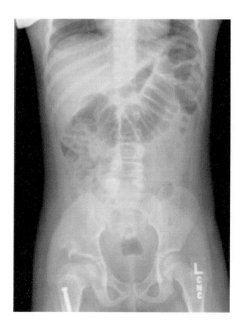

Figure 66.4 Abdominal x-ray Day 3.

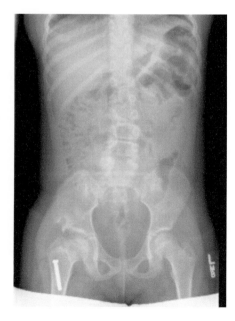

Figure 66.5 Abdominal x-ray Day 4.

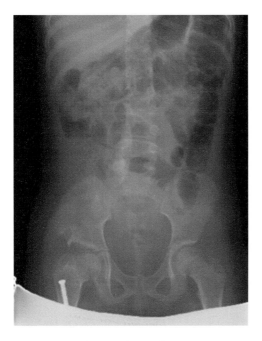

Figure 66.6 Abdominal x-ray day 5.

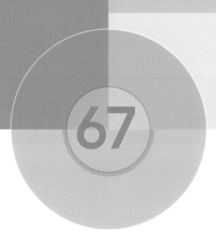
Bowel management program in a patient with prune belly syndrome: Case study

CASE HISTORY

- A 4-year-old boy with prune belly syndrome has chronic constipation.
- He is currently being managed with stool softeners. He is failing to empty his bowels, and soils daily.
- This patient has good potential for bowel control and he is mature enough to potty train as he has normal anatomy (normal anal sphincters, intact dentate line, and normal spine).
- Rectum appears dilated on contrast enema.
- There is no point of obstruction to suggest a stricture.

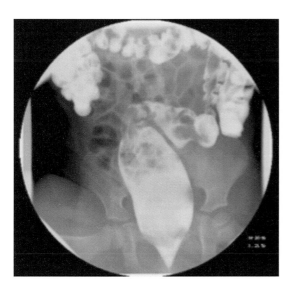

Figure 67.1 Contrast enema. What is your interpretation of the contrast enema? How would you manage his bowels (i.e., with laxatives or enemas)?

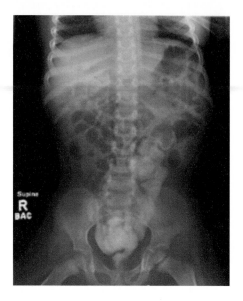

Figure 67.2 Bowel management radiographs. Day 1: Stool in the descending colon and rectum. Rectal enemas started given his age and maturity.

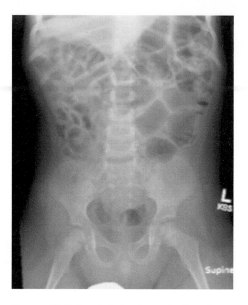

Figure 67.3 Day 2: Colon is empty. Rectal enema: 450 mL saline and 30 mL glycerin.

LEARNING POINTS

- This patient could be managed on laxatives or enemas.
- In our experience, children of this age are best managed with enemas in the first instance to get them clean and to increase their self-confidence.
- A future laxative trial can then be attempted when they are more mature and amenable to potty training. There is a significant psychological advantage to them once they "learn" what it is like to be clean from the mechanical emptying provided by the daily enema.

68

Constipation in a five-year-old girl: Case study

CASE HISTORY

- 5-year-old female, who presented to the emergency room with a history of abdominal pain, raising concern for appendicitis.
- Her abdominal ultrasound was negative but she continued to have non-specific symptoms.
- On further questioning, she was found to have urinary urgency, but no episodes of incontinence. She was also requiring stool softeners for constipation. She also noted some lower back pain.
- She underwent a magnetic resonance imaging scan and the findings are shown below.

REVIEW 68.1 MULTIPLE CHOICE QUESTION

What does this image show?

A. Enlarged bladder with stones
B. Pre-sacral mass
C. Appendix mass
D. Normal

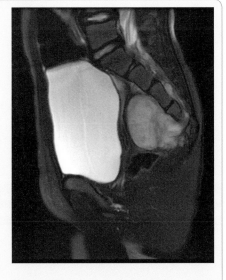

Figure 68.1 Lateral image of MRI.

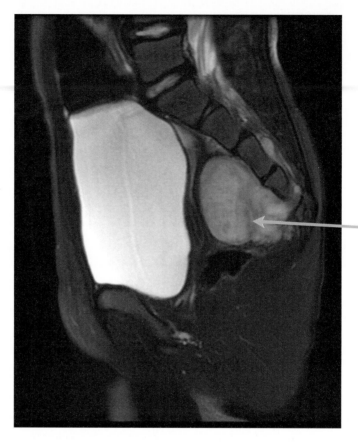

Figure 68.2 Magnetic resonance imaging scan of the spine and pelvis. Large pre-sacral mass originating from S3–S4 and S4–S5 foramina.

LEARNING POINTS

- This incidentally found mass, that explained the patient's non-specific symptoms, was approached through a posterior sagittal incision, with the rectum being dissected free to allow access to the tumor in collaboration with neurosurgery.
- It is important to assess all such pre-sacral masses for communication of the mass with the spinal cord.
- Histology confirmed this to be a ganglioneuroma.

ANSWER

68.1   B

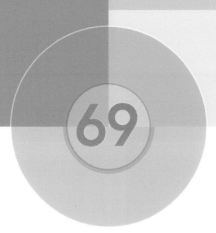

Surgical options following medical management failure: Case study

CASE HISTORY

- This is a case of a 13-year-old girl, with a long-standing history of constipation.
- Previous medical management has included high-dose laxatives without success.
- Cecostomy was placed and antegrade flushes were introduced without success (saline, bisacodyl, and glycerin).
- We decided to repeat a trial of laxatives because we felt that previously the laxative regimen was not aggressive enough—radiographs shown in Figure 69.4.

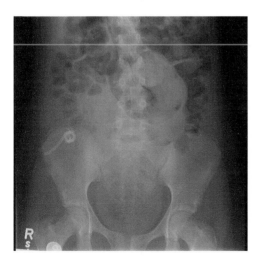

Figure 69.1 Bowel management radiographs. Day 1: loaded rectum. Given Fleet enema to clear the rectum. Cecostomy flush: 750 mL saline, 30 mL glycerin, and 27 mL soap.

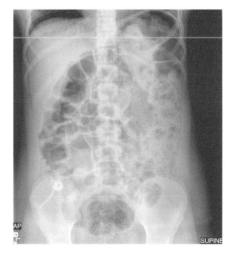

Figure 69.2 Stool in left colon.

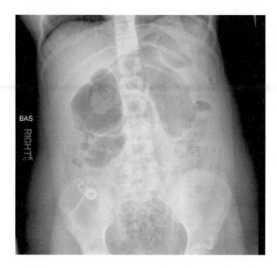

Figure 69.3 Stool in rectum.

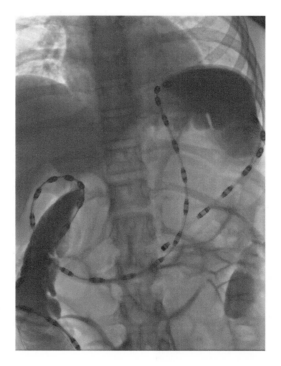

Figure 69.4 Colonic manometry catheter.

MANAGEMENT PLAN

- Patient once again failed medical management.
- Cecostomy flushes and high-dose laxatives are not clearing the colon.
- Patient was referred for motility studies.

RESULTS

- Study demonstrated that the distal 50–60 cm of the colon has abnormal motility, and redundancy of the sigmoid was seen on contrast enema.
- The right colon was also assessed with a manometry catheter placed via the cecostomy, demonstrating normal colonic motility in the ascending colon.

MANAGEMENT

- Laparoscopic resection of the distal colon (and the proximal rectum in a patient with functional/idiopathic constipation) with continued use of the cecostomy.

PLAN

- Careful adjustment of the cecostomy flushes
- Flush adjusted; currently 500 mL saline, 30 mL glycerin, and 9 mL Castile soap (poor response)
- Current regimen with 30-minute response
  - 500 mL saline
  - 30 mL glycerin

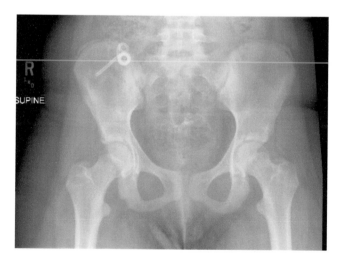

Figure 69.5 New regimen employed. X-ray is clean of stool and patient is clean.

LEARNING POINT

After colonic resection colon is easier to clean with antegrade flush regimen. In future (in 6–12 months), laxatives could be tried again and are expected to work at a much lower dose than has been tried previously.

70

Colonic motility evaluation: Case study

CASE HISTORY

- An 11-year-old girl with a history of chronic (functional) constipation.
- She has previously been managed on high-dose laxatives, which failed to resolve her symptoms.
- A cecostomy was placed and attempts were made to manage her with cecostomy flushes:
  - Saline 500 mL and glycerin 20 mL.
  - These were also unsuccessful.
- The antegrade cecostomy flushes also failed to empty the colon and she went on to have colonic motility studies.

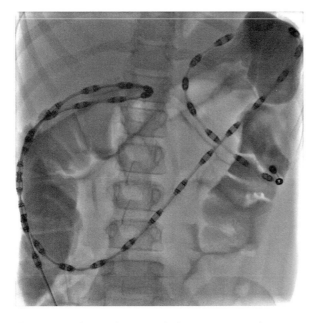

Figure 70.1 Image showing colonic manometry probe.

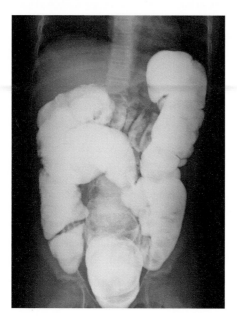

Figure 70.2 Contrast enema. Redundant dilated colon. Hepatic and splenic flexure noted to have more significant redundancy.

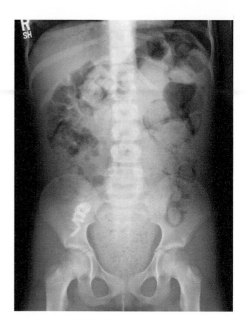

Figure 70.3 Plain abdominal radiograph. Despite hospitalization and monitored cecostomy flushes, the colon fails to empty.

COLONIC MANOMETRY

- No evidence of high-amplitude propagating contractions (HAPCs) seen after 5 mg bisacodyl.
- Patient passed several stools throughout the assessment, but these were not associated with any HAPCs.
- A second dose of bisacodyl was administered and there was no change in the response.

CONCLUSION

- Near total colonic inertia

ANORECTAL MANOMETRY

- Good squeeze pressure and normal resting pressure
- First balloon sensation 120 mL
- First urge to defecate 180 mL balloon
- Conclusion: Normal anorectal manometry

CONTRAST ENEMA: SEE FIGURE 70.2

- Redundant colon
- No evidence of stricture

What are your management options for this patient?

MANAGEMENT

- This child was noted to be failing to thrive. Her weight was plotted below the 3rd centile.
- The decision was made to manage this child with an ileostomy, to give the colon a period of time diverted. In the 4-month period post-ileostomy creation, she gained over 10 kg in weight.
- The future management plan is to repeat the colonic motility testing in 12 months and assess whether:
  - The colon has recovered following a period of being defunctioned, and she would be able to have the ileostomy closed.
  - The colon has failed to recover/continues to show abnormal motility and colonic resection. She would benefit from colonic resection of the abnormal segment.

LEARNING POINTS

Management options

- **Option 1:** Ileostomy and review colonic motility following period of bowel rest via the cecostomy. Can the ileostomy be reversed?
- **Option 2:** Colonic resection and continued use of the cecostomy flushes, but at reduced volume.
- **Option 3:** Colonic resection and revise the tube cecostomy to a Malone appendicostomy.

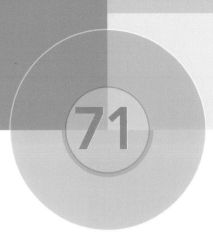

Bowel management— A problem related to the treatment: Case study

71

CASE HISTORY

- A 5-year-old boy with idiopathic constipation comes to your clinic for bowel management.
- Previous medical therapy has included lactulose, Miralax, senna, and bisacodyl, but he has continued to have soiling and accidents.
- During the bowel management week, he was recommenced on senna. After 2 days, he presents with inflammation and blistering to the groin and perineum.

Senna induce dermatitis is related to the additives in the senna, not the senna itself. Usually just changing the type of senna product that is used solves this problem.

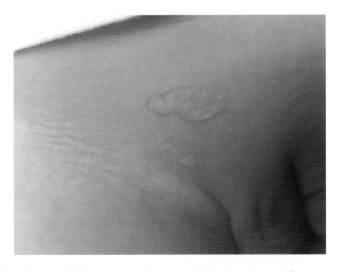

Figure 71.1 Clinical image. Blistering seen in the groin. What is the diagnosis?

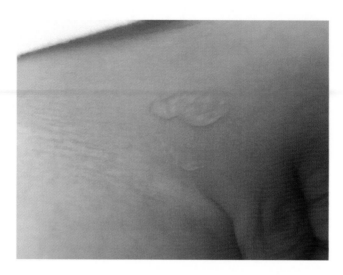

Figure 71.2 Senna-induced dermatitis (Leventhal JM et al. *Pediatrics* 2001; 107(1): 178–179; Smith WA et al. *Arch Dermatol* 2012; 148(3): 402–404).

REFERENCES

Leventhal JM et al. Laxative-induced dermatitis of the buttocks incorrectly suspected to be abusive burns. *Pediatrics* 2001; 107(1): 178–179.

Smith WA et al. Senna-containing laxative inducing blistering in toddlers. *Arch Dermatol* 2012; 148(3): 402–404.

Index